"With this book, mothers—*and* their helpers—can finally get breastfeeding right! A caring text, delightful illustrations, and clear, instructive pictures. Key positioning elements are shown to enable breastfeeding to proceed uneventfully, as an integral part of parenting—without fanfare, but with much love and good feelings."

Kathleen Auerbach, PhD
International Board Certified Lactation Consultant
University of Chicago Medical Center
Departments of Pediatrics and OB/GYN

"Wholeheartedly recommended by the Joint Breastfeeding Initiative, England."

Organizations in the Joint Breastfeeding Initiative
include the National Childbirth Trust, the Association
of Breastfeeding Mothers, and La Leche League (GB)

"Among the myriad 'how-to' books on breastfeeding, *Bestfeeding* delivers a uniquely rule-free, logical, and immensely practical guide to successful nursing. Great attention is focused on the 'mechanics' of breastfeeding, in particular the position of the baby and the latch onto the breast. Secondary problems, such as sore nipples, mastitis, and insufficient milk production, frequently have their origin in faulty mechanics. This valuable reference will enable mothers to avoid problems and enjoy their experience while they understand the simple and critical dynamics of the nursing process."

Jane Morton, MD, Pediatrician
Clinical Professor of Pediatrics
Stanford University Medical Center

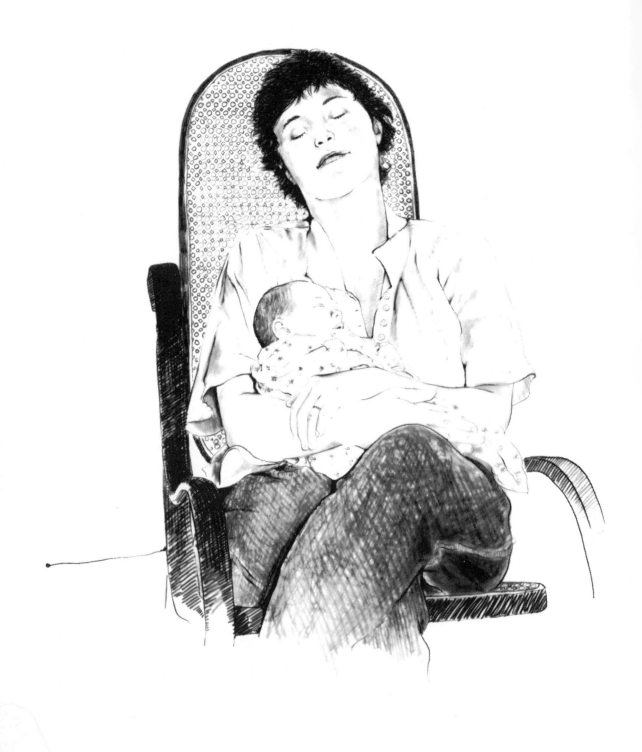

BESTFEEDING:

Getting Breastfeeding Right for You

An Illustrated Guide

BY

Mary Renfrew
Chloe Fisher
Suzanne Arms

CELESTIAL ARTS
Berkeley, California

Published by:
CELESTIAL ARTS
P.O. Box 7327
Berkeley, California 94707
United States of America

Cover photo by Suzanne Arms (aka Suzanne Arms Wimberley)
Cover and text design by Nancy Austin
Composition by Auto-Graphics, Inc.

Library of Congress Cataloging-in-Publication Data
    Renfrew, Mary, 1955–
        Bestfeeding : getting breastfeeding right for you : an illustrated guide / by Mary Renfrew, Chloe Fisher, and Suzanne Arms ; photos by Suzanne Arms ; illustrations by Maggie Conroy.
            p. cm.
        Bibliography: p.
        Includes index.
        ISBN 0-89087-571-5
        1. Breast feeding—Popular works. I. Fisher, Chloe, 1932–   . II. Arms, Suzanne. III. Conroy, Maggie. IV. Title.
    RJ216.R385 1989
    649'.33—dcl9   89–920
                                                                                CIP

First Printing, 1990

0   9   8   7   6   5   4   3   2

96   95   94   93   92   91   90

Manufactured in the United States of America

This book is dedicated
to all women
who have had problems with breastfeeding—
to those who struggled on despite difficulties,
and to those who gave up breastfeeding
before they wanted to.

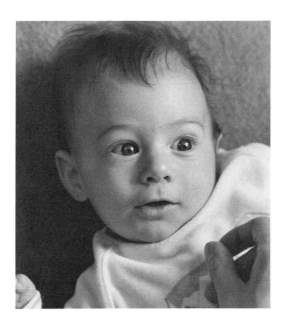

It is also dedicated with affection
and respect
to
Dr. Mavis Gunther,
whose work started us on the right road.

CONTENTS

ACKNOWLEDGMENTS

Like breastfeeding itself, this book needed support, and it benefited from the wisdom and guidance of skilled helpers. We were privileged to have the help of many people throughout the world in its preparation. The information we offer is based on clinical and personal experience, as well as a great deal of research. We are especially indebted to the work of Kathy Auerbach, Maureen Minchin and Mike Woolridge, whose understanding of breastfeeding and creativity in the field has contributed much to this book.

Most of what we have learned about breastfeeding has come from mothers, from fathers, and from babies. We want to acknowledge all the families we have worked with through the years. Our special thanks go to the women and families who allowed us to photograph them for this book: Sparrow Baranyai and Gary Blackburn, Martha Lopez-Chubb, Jackie and Larry Foreman, Christine Hunner, Judith Landry, Jenchyn and Raymond Luh, Lorri and Diego Roa, Lawan Jackson, Ann Marie Joyce, and Lesley Searle.

Many people read and commented on the text, and in so doing made it better. For correcting our errors, challenging our assumptions, and helping keep dogma to a minimum, we sincerely thank Kathy Auerbach, David Baum, Maggie Conroy, Donna Cowan, Susan Currie, Jo Garcia, Faye Gibson, Lynne Gleason, Karyn Kaufman, Brian McClelland, Kathy Michaelson, Maureen Minchin, Jane Morton, Gay Palmer, Harriet Palmer, and Mike Woolridge. Thank you, Barbara Henry and Shirley Anne Seel, for help with the resources section.

We believe we found the perfect illustrator for our book in Maggie Conroy. Thank you, Maggie, for your sensitive heart, discerning eye, and skillful hand.

Special thanks to Maria Tiscareño for the Spanish translation of concepts in the storyboard.

Our publishers believed in us and supported us all along the way in our efforts to create an inexpensive yet lavishly beautiful book. Thank you, David Hinds and Paul Reed at Celestial Arts. Thank you also to The Department of Health, England, which supported Mary Renfrew during the writing of this book, and to everyone at the National Perinatal Epidemiology Unit at Oxford for your understanding and practical support.

We have had lots of personal support as

well, from family and friends. All of them believed in and encouraged us, even when our work on this book got in the way of time they wanted to spend with us. A special thanks, John Wimberley, for allowing us to take over your home while we wrote, held meetings, and conducted interviews with breastfeeding mothers. Thanks for cups of tea and hugs, for making us laugh, and for giving us the brilliant title for this book.

Our own mothers were all strong women who wanted to breastfeed their babies but lived during times when breastfeeding was difficult. We are grateful for their perseverance in trying to do what was best for their children, and for their strong influence on our lives.

Some places too have been special to us in the creation of this book. Without a visit to Glastonbury, England, the book might never have been conceived. We worked together in Oxford, England, and in Palo Alto, California, and both of these places influenced our work, giving us the pleasure of long walks and magnificent skies.

More than anything, the joy of this book for us has been our collaboration with each other. Our different backgrounds, experiences, and ages have make our work together special, and we have learned a great deal from each other. For all of this we are most grateful.

ABOUT THIS BOOK

What This Book Contains

☆ *Breastfeeding is by far the best way to feed a baby. Most women know this. But breastfeeding is not always easy for women who live in societies where it is hidden, and we don't get a chance to learn how to do it. Some women find that breastfeeding is easy and satisfying, right from the start. But many women find it difficult to do without help, and it can be hard to find the right help.*

This book is about getting breastfeeding right for you and your baby, from the very beginning, and solving any problems quickly and easily.

There are many detailed photographs and illustrations that will show you exactly what to do. These pictures are probably the most valuable part of the book, as it is always easier to understand breastfeeding by seeing it than by reading about it.

The book has three important subjects: why breastfeeding is best for you; how to get the basics of breastfeeding right, including a simple checklist; breastfeeding problems: causes and solutions.

The same principles that help you get it right from the start will also guide you in treating common problems. Even unusual situations—which are rare in breastfeeding—can be improved or corrected by following these guidelines. If you have a special problem and need more help, there is a list of further, more detailed reading and a directory of good resources and organizations in different countries.

We give only information that we are confident about, and that has been well tried and tested. When we make observations and suggestions that are not yet fully supported by research, we point this out.

The reference list at the back of the book gives what we feel are some of the most significant sources in the huge volume of literature used in the preparation of this book. The index will help you find what you need quickly.

Three practical points:

1. We have written this book so that it is appropriate for all those who read English. There are cultural differences in the use and writing of the English language. With one English, one American, and one Scottish author who has spent part of her life in Canada, we hope we have achieved a balance of language. We have chosen one consistent style of spelling. Because our publisher is American, we use American spelling throughout. We hope that non-Americans do not feel excluded by this.

2. Babies are either girls or boys. We acknowledge this by alternating the use of *him* and *her*, *she* and *he* in different sections of the book.

3. We are using the term *health worker* to include every trained person a woman may have access to—professional or lay, licensed or not. Where we mean specifically a medical practitioner, we say so.

What This Book Will Do for You

☆ *This book will help you get the basics of breastfeeding right, for you and for your baby. It will help you to prevent problems and treat them quickly if they occur.*

What we offer does not include the use of drugs or mechanical interventions, such as nipple shields or the regular use of bottles. We do mention a few simple aids, such as spoons, cups, and breast pumps, for use in special situations. Our main purpose, however, is to show you the basics of breastfeeding, which require only you and your baby. Most of the problems women have are a result of not knowing these basic principles. You can often work out your own problems if you have the right information. Some problems will need specialist help, but all mothers and babies need to understand the basics first.

This book will help others help you to continue with good breastfeeding. Sometimes it is hard to solve problems on your own. You can share this book with your partner, your helpers, or others who are important to you. It will help them to support you! Many people say it is hard to support breastfeeding when someone they care for is struggling with problems, is exhausted, or is in pain. Understandably they want to take action to help. Sadly, the most common remedy today is to give the baby a bottle, rather than try to solve the real problem.

This book will help you to avoid and understand the conflicting advice so commonly given to women. It may contradict much of what you have heard (and may well continue to hear) from family, friends, and health workers. There are reasons for this, which we will explain. *This book will help you to sort out the good advice from the bad.*

 This book will give you back a real choice in feeding your baby: *the choice to breastfeed well, with pleasure, by avoiding problems or solving them early and successfully. We want every woman to be able to say what one mother recently said about her baby daughter: "She's been a joy—for all of us!"*

Who This Book Is For

This book is for all women, all over the world, who want to know more about feeding their babies. It is for you.

- Whether you have or have not yet decided to breastfeed

- Whether you have or have not yet had a baby

- Whether you are having your first baby, or your second, third, or fourth

- Whether you have or have not had feeding problems in the past

- Whether you are having one baby, twins, or more

- Whether you are on your own or surrounded by friends and helpers

- Whether you are aged fourteen or forty

It is also for people who want to help, such as:

- Men who want to help but are not sure how

- Family and friends who want to offer their support

- Health workers and their students, who work with women and babies

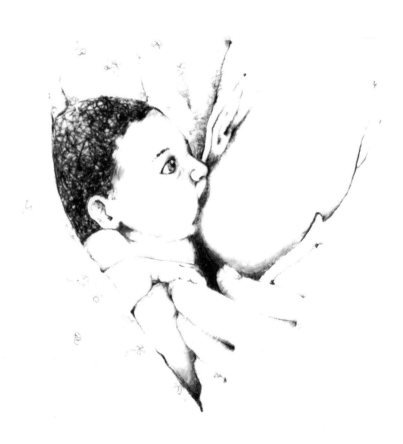

Why Women Want to Breastfeed

We do not pretend to be unbiased. Like most women, we believe that breastfeeding is the best way to feed a baby. The evidence is that breastfeeding is good for mothers and babies, and no other form of infant feeding has yet been devised that does not have drawbacks.

Best for Babies

Most people know that breast milk is the best nourishment for babies. It is perfectly balanced with protein, fat, minerals, and vitamins. And it even changes its composition throughout the day, and over the months, to suit each baby. Most people also know that breastfeeding is the best possible protection against infection and disease. In fact, the more we learn about breastfeeding, the more advantages we see for the baby and the mother.

In many parts of the world the difference between breastfeeding and bottle feeding is the difference between life and death. Even in countries where bottle feeding is safe, there are still disadvantages.

For example, it has been shown that breastfeeding is good for:

- The efficiency of the baby's immune system

- The strength of the mother–child relationship

- The eating habits of babies, children, and even adults who have been breastfed

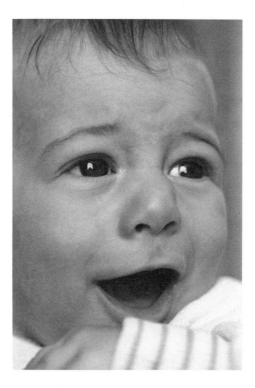

Breastfeeding is best for babies.

Breastfeeding also seems to decrease the chances of children developing allergies, cancer, and other problems such as coeliac disease in later life. Adults who have been breastfed seem to be less likely to develop arteriosclerosis, and if it does occur, it is likely to be less severe. This area is difficult to research, and studies give few definitive answers. But there are strong indications that these things are true.

There are also some studies that suggest that breastfeeding may be good for brain development, for healing the effects of trauma at birth, for children's interpersonal relationships, for children's ability to give comfort and to comfort themselves, and for children's sleeping patterns. *Artificial feeding provides none of these unique protections. And even in Western countries, babies who are fed artificially have a higher hospital admission rate than babies who are breastfed, especially those who are fully breastfed.*

New information from research done in Sweden suggests that hormones in the baby's digestive system are released by suckling. These hormones help to stimulate the baby's growth and to calm her too. Not only are you feeding your baby, but you are helping her grow and keeping her calm and happy.

Best for Women

Breastfeeding is not only best for babies. It affects women too. Just as in pregnancy it is impossible to separate the mother and baby, so in breastfeeding their physical and emotional welfare are interconnected. A baby who is breastfeeding well is content and grows steadily, and his mother will therefore be more relaxed and happy. Similarly, a relaxed and happy mother is more likely to be able to care well for her baby than an anxious and distressed mother.

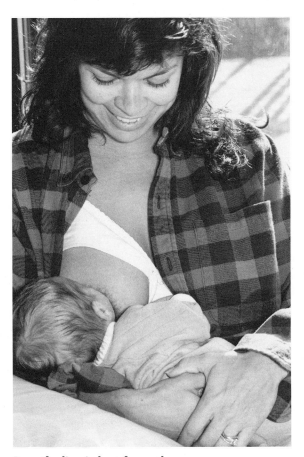

Breastfeeding is best for mothers.

For example, women find that when they breastfeed:

- Their wombs contract more quickly after birth.

- The blood loss after childbirth (lochia) flows faster and is completed more quickly.

- They are less likely to become pregnant again soon after birth, especially when breastfeeding is frequent and prolonged.

- The hormones they secrete while breastfeeding make them feel calm.

- The hormones make their bodies more efficient while breastfeeding; they don't have to "eat for two," because their bodies conserve energy and use stored energy instead.

- They lose weight more easily, especially around the thighs and buttocks, where fat is usually so hard to shift.

- In later life women who have breastfed seem to be less likely to develop cancer of the breasts, ovaries, or cervix. More research is needed to confirm these effects.

Best for Families

Mothers say that breastfeeding gives them quiet, relaxing times together with their babies throughout the day. If breastfeeding works well, it is pleasurable for mother and baby, and is good for the way a mother and her child feel about themselves and about each other.

Breastfeeding is far more than a way to feed a baby. It is a time when babies and mothers give and receive love. Babies respond not just to the breast milk they take in, but also to the skin-to-skin contact that occurs. Often, crying and distressed babies are comforted by this cuddly contact.

The repeated positive feelings of nurturing and physical closeness are the best possible foundation for a good relationship between mother and baby, and for building the confidence and self-esteem of both. This, in turn, will help promote the development of healthy relationships within the whole family.

Best for Women and Babies
with Special Needs

Breastfeeding is best for women and babies, even in special situations, such as having twins or triplets. A woman can produce enough milk to feed more than one baby, and it is often possible to feed two babies at once, once breastfeeding each baby is well established. Many women who must live in circumstances that are far from ideal have discovered breastfeeding to be one thing from which they can draw comfort and support. Breastfeeding well can help a woman gain the confidence to deal with even very difficult circumstances in her life, whether they are physical difficulties or emotional ones.

When the baby needs extra special care, breastfeeding can also help there. It is always hard for parents with small, sick, or premature babies to feel fully involved in their care while they are in the hospital. A

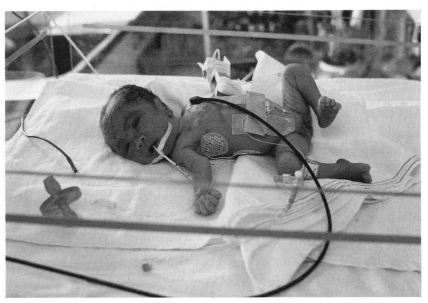

Breastfeeding is best for babies with special needs. Babies who are very small or sick need both the benefits of breast milk and the warm, close contact breastfeeding provides.

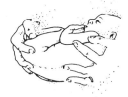

mother who expresses her breast milk, and then puts her baby to the breast when she can, is giving her baby a special gift that no one else can. A woman will often say that it involves her in her baby's care and gives her a closeness to her baby that nothing else could.

Studies have looked at the benefits of skin-to-skin contact between mothers and their small or sick babies. Often this contact involves the baby nuzzling, or actually feeding, at the breast. Mothers who do this are likely to continue to breastfeed longer than mothers who have not had this opportunity. Their babies gain weight faster and go home from the hospital sooner than do babies fed artificial milk.

Balancing the Benefits and Problems

For each woman, the decision to breast or to bottle feed is a balance between a number of factors. Sometimes these factors conflict. For example, you might believe that breastfeeding is best for your baby, but your sister had serious problems breastfeeding and you are worried the same might happen to you. Or perhaps you want to breastfeed, but you also need, or want, to go back to work soon after your baby's birth. Maybe you are worried about information you have heard about contamination of breast milk due to pollution in our environment. You worry that this might harm your baby, yet, otherwise, you know that breastfeeding is best for your baby.

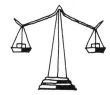

Think carefully and weigh the benefits against the hazards before you make a decision. In almost every case, breastfeeding will be by far the best way to feed your baby, and often it will be best for you too. But you need to think through the things that worry you.

Will Breastfeeding Be Difficult for You?

You cannot know this in advance. But the best thing to do is exactly what you are doing: learn as much as you can, find good help, and then try to breastfeed. Some women have no problems, and most problems that do occur can be treated. This book will help you prevent many of the common problems and provides effective solutions if they do arise.

Can You Combine Breastfeeding and Working? (see also page 155)

Yes, you can. It is not easy in societies where the workplace is separated from the home, but it can be done. The more time you can be together with your baby during the first few months, the better for both of you. The best preparation for going back to work is to be breastfeeding without problems. If you have problems *and* go back to work, it is much harder to keep breastfeeding. Whatever happens, and whenever you go back to work, remember that breastfeeding for even a short time is better for both of you than not breastfeeding at all.

It helps a lot to be in touch with other women who have combined working outside the home with breastfeeding. The challenge can be managed in many different ways. You will get ideas about what may work for you by talking with women who have done it.

Think carefully about all the possibilities. The time you spend thinking creatively and planning carefully ensures that you and your baby can have the solution that is best for you both.

Can you take paid maternity leave? If not, are you in a position to take unpaid leave, even for a short while? Can you find good child care close to your workplace, where you could feed at lunchtime? Can your husband or partner take a few months off work and bring the baby to you for feeding at lunchtime? Can you take your baby to work? (If you have a sympathetic employer and colleagues, this is not as impossible as it sounds. In the first few months, many babies simply feed and then sleep quietly.) Can you work part-time for a while? Can you arrange for the time and a quiet place at work to express your milk? Can you arrange to job share? This would mean finding someone to work half-time at your job. One of you could work mornings and the other could work afternoons, or each could work two-and-a-half days a week. Some women who job share look after each others' baby during the time the other is at work.

If none of these solutions are possible, then you might think about cutting down on breastfeeding. The person caring for your baby can give bottles of expressed breast milk or of formula while you are away. You can breastfeed in the evenings and on weekends. It is perfectly possible to breastfeed two or three times a day for as long as you want. (See page 155 for more about breastfeeding and working.)

QUESTIONS TO ASK
ABOUT GOING BACK TO WORK

☐ Can I take paid maternity leave?

☐ If not, can I take unpaid leave, even for a short while?

☐ Can I work part-time for a while?

☐ Can I find good child care close to my workplace?

☐ Can I breastfeed at lunchtime or on coffee breaks?

☐ Can I take my baby to work for a while?

☐ Can my partner take time off work and arrange to bring the baby to me for feeding?

☐ Can I arrange for the time and a quiet place at work to express my milk?

Don't forget you can breastfeed in the evenings and on weekends, while the person caring for your baby feeds expressed breast milk or formula.

What About Contaminants?

In recent years newspaper and magazine articles and radio and television programs have warned about the contamination of breast milk by substances such as pesticides and other chemicals. Some women have chosen not to breastfeed as a result of this information.

In fact, in many cases, the contamination of cow's milk, which is the basis of almost all alternative feeds for babies, is worse than the contamination of breast milk. A thorough report on dioxins in the environment (the chemicals that give most cause for concern) from the U.K. states that the known advantages of breastfeeding outweigh the possible risks at present. The solution to this problem is seldom to stop breastfeeding, which would mean the baby would lose all the health-giving aspects of breast milk too. The solution is to be aware of the problem and to avoid as many sources of contamination as possible. In the long term we need to work toward preventing and clearing up the pollution that caused the contamination in the first place—using lead-free fuel, changing industrial processes such as incineration and paper bleaching, and finding alternatives to stubble burning are all important.

The World Health Organization has been working on this problem for some years, and there are some indications that the situation regarding pollution that affects breast milk may be improving overall.

One final note: It is clear from research that breast milk does not contain high levels of minerals such as lead and aluminum, which are found in some modern formulas and in some nations' water supplies and which can cause brain damage.

Human Immunodeficiency Virus and AIDS

In the past few years, there has been concern about the risk of babies becoming infected by the human immunodeficiency virus (HIV) through breastfeeding. HIV is the virus that causes acquired immune deficiency syndrome (AIDS). There is still no cure for AIDS, and it is important that babies are protected as much as possible from infection.

HOW IS THE VIRUS TRANSMITTED?

HIV lives in body fluids such as blood, semen, and vaginal secretions. HIV can be passed from someone who has the virus during sexual intercourse or by the sharing of injection needles. It can also be passed from a mother who has the virus to her unborn baby in pregnancy, and this is the most common way in which babies become infected.

Receiving treatment with blood and blood products, such as by blood transfusion or during treatment for hemophilia (a disease that causes problems with blood clotting), is a possible source of infection. In many countries, however, blood donations are now screened for the virus, and blood products are treated to ensure that if HIV or other viruses are present, they are inactivated.

Remember that other forms of contact with a person who has the virus, such as touching or kissing, will not put you at risk of infection.

HIV can persist in the body for several years without causing disease, and many people do not know that they have it. If you are concerned that you may have the virus, then talk to a health worker. You may even want to have a blood test.

IS HIV TRANSMITTED IN BREAST MILK?

We still know very little about whether HIV is transmitted from mothers to babies in breast milk. At the time this book went to print (February 1990), there are reports of a *very small number* of babies in the world who *may* have become infected in this way. These babies were fed either by:

- Mothers who became infected after the birth of their baby by a transfusion with blood that had not been tested and was infected with HIV or

- Wet nurses who were ill with AIDS

In both of these situations, the milk *might* be especially infective. These cases are quite unusual.

BALANCING THE RISKS AND BENEFITS

It may be possible, probably in exceptional circumstances, for HIV to be transmitted in breast milk. Many babies have been fed by infected, but healthy, mothers and have not become infected themselves. The risks and the benefits of breastfeeding must be balanced. Deciding not to breastfeed means that the baby will not receive the advantages of breastfeeding and the important properties of breast milk, including protection from infection. These benefits are especially important in countries where alternatives to breastfeeding are not safe.

Choosing to Breastfeed

Despite the fact that most women know that breastfeeding is best for their babies, some decide not to breastfeed, and others stop after a short time. When we look at some of the problems that women face when feeding their babies, this is not hard to understand.

A woman who chooses not to breastfeed always has reasons for doing so, which usually include:

- Breastfeeding does not appeal to her or is distasteful to her.

- She believes that breastfeeding is inconvenient and that bottle feeding is a good substitute, and much easier.

- She plans to go back to work outside the home soon after the baby is born and feels it is too difficult to work and also breast-feed.

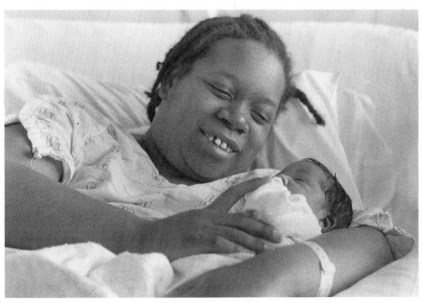

Many women look forward to breastfeeding as a time of special closeness with their babies and something only they can give.

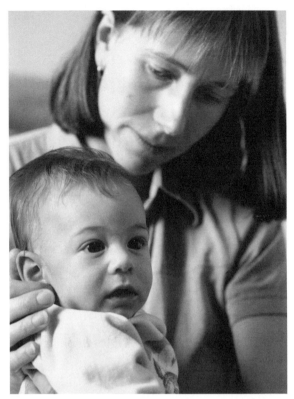

Some women feel a bit anxious at the idea of breastfeeding. This may be because of things others
have said or negative experiences they have had.

When a woman finds the idea of breastfeeding unappealing, it may
be a result of her own or other people's experiences, or it may be because
she associates breastfeeding with something distasteful. She may, for
example, be shy about exposing her breasts or dislike her body. But
women in cultures where modesty is prized breastfeed, even in public
places, without exposing their breasts. And many women who have
learned to dislike or distrust their bodies, but who have been willing to
breastfeed for all the benefits it has for their babies, have found a measure of comfort and pleasure in breastfeeding they had never thought
possible.

A woman who decides not to breastfeed because she believes bottle
feeding is equal to breastfeeding and easier is usually unaware of the
difficulties, hazards, and practical drawbacks of bottle feeding.

A woman who plans to go back to work outside the home while her baby is very young and believes it is not possible both to do this and to breastfeed needs information that it is possible to do both, for her own benefit and for her baby's.

Some women today, because of their experience and the attitudes of those around them, believe that breastfeeding will not suit their ways of life. They believe that bottle feeding is a good choice for themselves and their babies.

It is important that every woman make a free choice about how to feed her baby. She cannot do this unless she has full information about breastfeeding and bottle feeding, breast milk and artificial milk. A woman who chooses not to breastfeed might want to ask herself, Why do I not want to breastfeed? Are my reasons sound? Can some of the problems be overcome?

If women found breastfeeding easy, *if* our culture did not lead some women to regard the workings of their bodies with uneasiness, and *if* artificial substitutes were not so heavily advertised and easily available, *then* women would truly have free choice.

 Women are often prevented from doing what they would like to do by three things:

1. **Misinformation** they are given by others, which creates bad habits and leads to breastfeeding problems

2. **Lack of skilled support**, especially in the first days and weeks

3. **Practical difficulties** they can't solve

You can see that the problems of breastfeeding, which are common, arise largely from social, not individual, causes.

It is not a woman's fault if she chooses not to breastfeed, or if she stops in the first weeks or months. It is often the fault of the culture in which we live. Women are simply not being given the accurate information and skilled support they need to carry on.

Some cultures look on breasts mainly for sexual pleasure, and women often find it hard to expose their breasts to feed their babies (in spite of the fact that breastfeeding often exposes less of the breast than normal beachwear). Many men in Western society also find it hard for their partners to breastfeed while other people are around. Some even feel jealous and threatened by the special closeness their babies have with their mothers at their mothers' breasts. This is hard to deal with, because

A Formula for Trouble

TRY ADDING TOGETHER
a difficult-to-cope-with, unhappy baby
　　　(a common result of difficult breastfeeding)

WITH
a new mother who feels unsure of how to care for a baby
　　　(what new mother who has little experience of
　　　babies and little support from experienced
　　　mothers isn't unsure of herself?)

WITH
the demands of an already tiring life
　　　(what parent of a young child isn't usually tired
　　　and often dealing with long hours of work
　　　in or away from the home?)

AND YOU GET
the perfect recipe for breastfeeding failure!

ADD TO THAT
the fact that many women today are single parents
　　　(trying valiantly to do alone what traditionally
　　　was the job of a large, extended family)

PLUS
the fact that much advice women get
is inaccurate or discouraging

PLUS
the unease some people feel with breasts and breastfeeding
　　　(and it's hard not to feel this, given our culture's
　　　obsession with breasts as sex objects)

AND YOU GET *a sense of the seriousness*
and widespread nature of the problem.

the feelings are so deep rooted. It is a fact, however, that babies need breasts, and they need them to be available whenever they are hungry, not just when it is convenient for older people.

Women should not feel guilty for choosing to avoid or to solve their problems by bottle feeding. Sadness or anger might be more natural responses, for women have not had the help they need to learn and maintain this essential skill.

☆ *Successful breastfeeding must become a real choice for women today.* When it does many more people will gain confidence in the fact that women's bodies work, and that babies are the best judges of their own food intake.

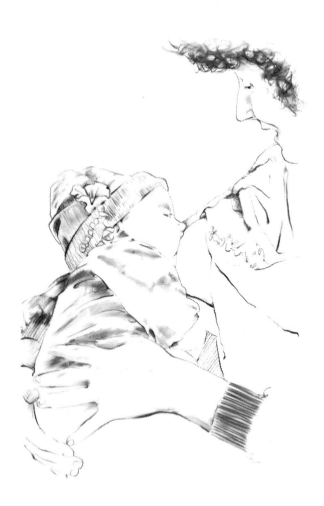

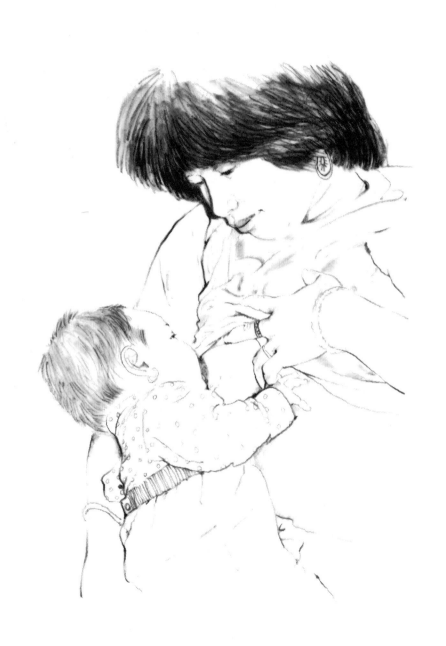

Starting to Breastfeed: Getting the Basics Right

Before You Begin—Finding Helpers

 Finding good helpers is one of the most important things you can do. It might also be one of the hardest.

All women who breastfeed their new babies can benefit from help, especially in the first three to four weeks. Even if you find breastfeeding easy from the beginning, you will need help to allow you time apart from the baby to catch up on your sleep. Whether this is your first baby or your sixth, you need to think about who is going to help you. Try to choose your helpers before your baby is born.

Note: If you don't have good support, this does not mean you will fail, or that you should choose to bottle feed. But it helps enormously to have assistance.

You will need three things from your helpers:

1. *Good emotional support* on an ongoing basis while you work on getting breastfeeding established or on solving problems

2. *Real practical help* with household tasks, such as shopping, cooking, cleaning, and caring for your older children

3. *Skilled assistance* if you have difficulty getting it right or if you develop problems

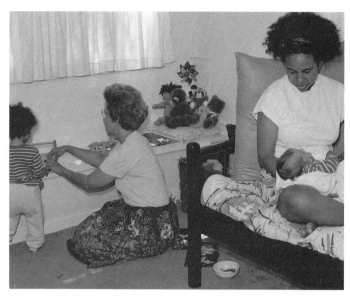

A helper can take care of the house, cook, and assist with older children. She can make things a lot easier for you, so that you can concentrate on getting breastfeeding established and enjoying your baby.

Helpers can be your friends, husband or partner, family, doctor, midwife, nurse, lactation consultant, or breastfeeding support group. Women who have breastfed well or a nutritionist may also be able to help. If you cannot find good help, look at the resources listed at the back of this book. These organizations may be able to put you in touch with good help nearby.

Before you turn to someone for help, make sure whoever you ask is as interested in breastfeeding as you are. If one of his or her first solutions is to try bottle feeding, that person is not the right person to ask. If this happens to you, find someone else.

It is possible that one person alone (even the most loving and attentive husband or partner) will not be able to help you in every way necessary. It is unlikely that he or she will be available every time you need someone or be skilled at solving a physical problem, such as the position of the baby at the breast. But this person's emotional encouragement will be a great help, and together you may be able to resolve the problem or find additional help.

Usually a partner, friends, and family are good sources of help for emotional and practical support. You might want to ask your mother, another relative who supports your breastfeeding, or a friend to stay for the first few days to help.

If you ask someone to come and stay and help, then let him or her do just that. Don't be tempted to look after that person as a guest. And don't let him or her play with the baby while you do the dishes, either. This time is for you and your baby to get to know each other. Ask only someone you feel very relaxed with (and this may not necessarily be your mother, no matter how much she loves you).

Remember that because bottle feeding was common until the past few years, many older women did not breastfeed. Your mother and your mother-in-law may have bottle fed. Some will not be supportive of breastfeeding, simply because their experience was different. Do think carefully before you decide where to turn for help. The last thing you need to hear as you work on getting breastfeeding right at 2:00 A.M. is, "Why don't we just try a bottle?"

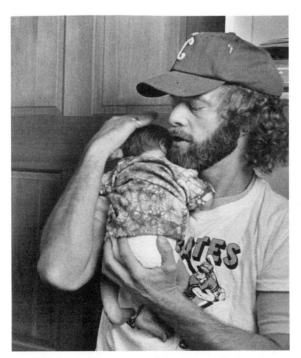

The father can be a tremendous help with the new baby and your greatest support during the first weeks, as you both learn to cope with little sleep and adjust your lives to this new person who needs so much care and attention.

If your partner is not supportive, then ask a friend you see often or who lives nearby to help. A woman who has breastfed well herself is an invaluable resource. A mother-to-mother support group, such as La Leche League, the National Childbirth Trust, or the Nursing Mothers Association of Australia, can often provide this sort of support. See the listing of resources at the back of the book for how to contact them.

A Word About Fathers

The father of your baby can be your best support for breastfeeding. He may enjoy watching and helping you and the baby be physically close and loving. Or he may find it challenging and uncomfortable, and he may feel left out or threatened by how close you and the baby are.

Because of the complex issues of sexuality and breastfeeding in many cultures, some men have ambivalent feelings about breastfeeding,

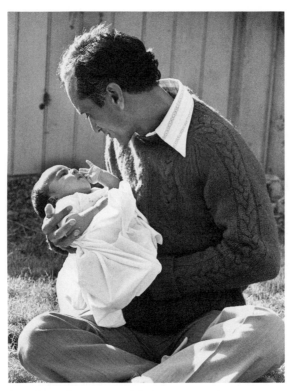

Sometimes the greatest help you can get is some time alone without your baby. A father also needs times alone with his baby.

of which they may not even be aware. Your baby's father may want to support you, yet find it hard when you need to feed in front of other people. He may like the idea of breastfeeding, but find the practicalities hard to take. Or he may be supportive while it is going well, but find it hard to watch you get sore and tired if you have problems.

It will be helpful if your husband or partner understands that in spite of the cultural attitudes that are not always supportive of breast-feeding, it is by far the best thing for your baby and for you. In the long run it will also be the best thing for him, as his baby will be healthier and family relationships will be better and stronger.

Some men say they want to feed their babies from the bottle so that they can share in feeding too. They need to understand that doing this in the early weeks could undermine the success of breastfeeding. They also need to know that artificial milk is not as good for a baby as breast milk (and it's more expensive).

Men can share in many ways, but feeding is best left to mothers and babies. Fathers can cuddle, comfort, bathe, and change babies, and they can enjoy watching you feeding the baby. They can have lots of loving contact, but they can't breastfeed.

Finding Skilled Assistance

Finding skilled assistance might be difficult because of the reasons dis-cussed on pages 157–159. Many health workers do not really under-stand breastfeeding, even if they are supportive. So be creative if you need to, and be persistent.

All the guidelines we have given in this section about finding help also apply to finding professional help. You might also want to talk to other women, and find out who has been helpful to them.

If there is no one nearby who has real skill, then find a health worker who is concerned and supportive, and take a copy of this book with you. Together you should be able to work it out.

Taking Care of Yourself

Having a new baby is likely to be the most demanding experience you will ever have. Along with discovering the real rewards and joys of this time, you will find that you are very tired. This is due in part to the inevitable nights of broken sleep and early waking.

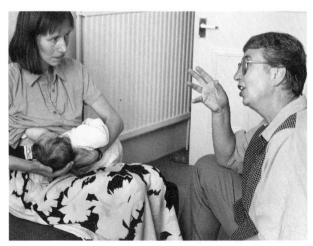

Make sure the person you choose to help you breastfeed is interested in breastfeeding and will take the time to work with you and your baby.

Don't be surprised that you don't have as much energy as you are used to. Most of your energy is going toward caring for your baby. This experience is valuable and rewarding, but you might find that you cannot work, at home or at your job, with the same enthusiasm as you did before. You now have an extra, time-consuming job to do, and your life will have to change.

Some magazines and books will tell you that you can still do it all—the Superwoman myth. This is not true. You might be able to do it for a while, but in the long term your own health and the happiness of those around you will suffer. Find ways of cutting back the other demands in your life, at least for a while. Doing less housework, or getting help with the basic tasks, is one way of adjusting. Many couples find that work in the home must be shared more evenly once they have a baby.

Make sure that you take some time for yourself at least once a day. Having someone care for your baby for a short time while you take a restful bath or walk or read quietly can make all the difference.

Everything you do for your baby, especially the things you do often in a day, such as picking her up, feeding her, changing her nappy or diaper, teaches your baby about you and her world. She learns about the world mostly from your behavior, through your touch and the feeling of love and care you give her. This makes it all the more important to take good care of yourself and to *treat yourself as if you are very special and worthwhile, because you are.*

How Breastfeeding Really Works: The Basics

 Breastfeeding without problems depends on getting the physical aspects right. Ideally, this means getting it right from the very first feed.

We will describe, and show you in photographs and drawings, exactly how to go about getting breastfeeding right.

We define breastfeeding as right if it is free of problems for you and your baby. We do not intend the word *right* to imply that there is only one way to breastfeed or that you have failed if you encounter difficulties. There are as many ways of breastfeeding as there are mothers and babies, and you will develop your own style, just as you would if you were dancing; but you need to know the steps first before you can add your own variations.

It is usually not difficult to get breastfeeding right—in fact, you and your baby may find it really easy—but you will need a bit of practice,

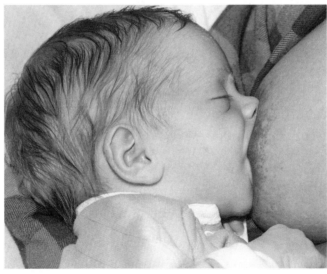

This baby, one of twins, was having difficulty at the breast until his mother learned how to get positioning just right. His brother, who was larger at birth, had no trouble; but like many small babies, positioning was critical for this little boy.

Here, at 3½ weeks, he is on the breast well for the very first time. His mother remarked on the difference in his behavior (he was much happier!) after just this one good feed.

and you may need the help and support of other people. Remember that many problems last only a week or two, and then you and your baby can go on to enjoy months of satisfying breastfeeding.

Some people may think it is unnecessary to go into such detail on these points. But women today didn't learn about breastfeeding by seeing it while growing up. Few older women know how to do it right. Many health professionals have never learned the techniques of breastfeeding. Most of us need to relearn the practicalities of breastfeeding. Maybe in thirty or forty years' time, so many women will have learned about breastfeeding that a book to teach the techniques will be unnecessary; but that time is not yet with us.

Remember that you will need practice to get it right. Think about how you learned to walk. It took practice and time; you didn't get it together all at once. You were clumsy at first. You fell sometimes. But you didn't criticize yourself because you didn't get it right the first time! You simply kept practicing, and one day you discovered you could do it easily.

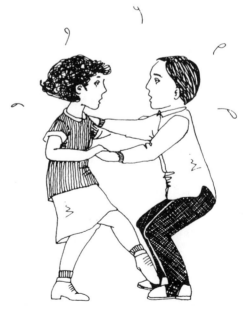

Like learning to dance, breastfeeding takes practice and rhythm because there are two of you doing it together.

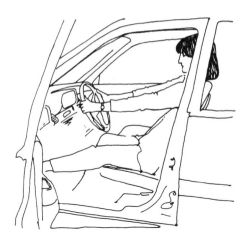

As in learning to drive a car,
positioning is *very* important.

Breastfeeding is a combination of instinct, reflex, and learning. For instance, you have an instinct to put your baby to your breast, and your baby has a reflex to open her mouth. Beyond that, you have to learn what to do with your breasts and your baby, and your baby has to learn what to do with her mouth and jaws.

It's like dancing: the two of you may like each other and like the rhythm of the music, but not know the steps to the dance. At first you may get tangled up every time you try, and have to laugh at yourselves. But once you get it right, you are a single unit: you move smoothly, without having to think about it, like one body. And although it can be difficult to learn, it is often fun to practice.

Or breastfeeding can be compared to learning to drive a car. You have to get all the details right, in the right sequence, before you can go anywhere without stalling constantly.

It will pay off if you take time and pay careful attention until breast-feeding is going smoothly. When you have learned to drive or to dance, you often wonder what all the fuss was about—but without the fuss, you probably never would have got it right. Once breastfeeding is established, without problems, it will be easy to enjoy both your baby *and* the rest of your life.

Simple does not always mean easy. What we offer is simple, but it may take time. Once you and your baby get it right, however, you will never forget it. You will add your own variations as you get more confident and as your baby grows, just as you do in developing your own style of dancing or driving.

You can use the information we provide here whether you are starting from your first feed or working on solving problems.

The basic principles we describe are the same at all stages of breast-feeding and for mothers and babies of all ages (although they are most important in the early days and weeks), and whether you are having your first or your fourth baby. They are also the same if you have more than one baby to feed or if your baby is small or sick or active or passive.

You will need to prepare for feeding. Quiet surroundings are very helpful for the first two weeks, as you and your baby learn about each other. Some women find that during this time they are easily distracted by visitors with whom they are not entirely comfortable, or even by the

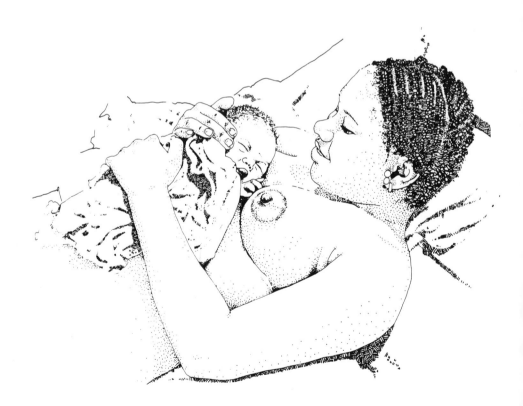

radio or television. Others find that putting on some calming music helps. Once you are quiet and comfortable, focus on your baby, not on what is going on around you.

Take the time you need to get breastfeeding right at the start; it will be easier later if you do. If you can arrange to have extra help in the house at this time, from your husband or partner, family member, or close friend, then do. But make sure it is someone with whom you feel comfortable; otherwise the help will cause more problems than it is worth. And don't be too worried about keeping the house tidy for a while. A happy, healthy baby and a few precious moments of quiet for yourself are more important than a tidy house.

Breastfeeding Your Baby for the First Time

 Breastfeeding for the first time—in fact, for the first few days or weeks, until it is easy—is best done when you, your baby, your partner, and your helpers are all calm.

Getting feeding right needs patience and quiet surroundings. It is good to feed soon after delivery, but it does not have to happen *immediately*. In fact, many babies and many mothers are not ready to feed right after birth; they both need time to adjust to what has just happened. Hold your baby close after birth if you can, and let her nuzzle at your breasts. If she is eager to feed, she will try to do so. If not, don't try to persuade her until you have calm, quiet time and help to get it right.

After a normal birth, it is probably best to wait until after your placenta is out, your stitches are done (if you need any), and you can move more freely. This will probably be within the first hour after birth. In the meantime, you can keep your baby in your arms and concentrate on enjoying her; you needn't think about breastfeeding until you have a bit of quiet and privacy. When you are ready to breastfeed her, ask for the help of a midwife, nurse, or family member.

Remember that both you and your baby have just worked very hard, and your bodies will need to recover. Many women like to lie down for the first feed, especially if they have stitches from an episiotomy or have had a cesarean. Some babies will be sleepy and need

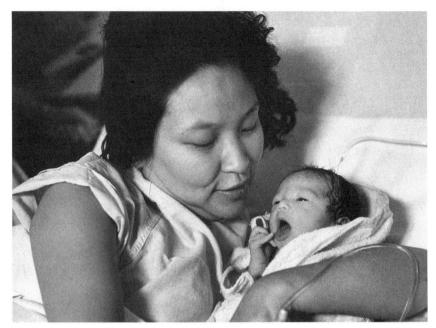

After a cesarean birth you can cuddle and hold your baby almost immediately.
Do ask for help to breastfeed for the first few times.

encouragement to feed for the first days, especially if they are small or
if their mothers were given medication in labor.

After an epidural or spinal anesthetic, you will still be awake and able
to hold your baby. After a spinal, you may need to lie flat for a few hours
to prevent a severe headache.

If you have had a cesarean section, you can still cuddle and feed your
baby soon after delivery, though you will need help. You will have to lie
in bed for the first hours, but will probably be encouraged to get up and
move around soon after, to promote healing.

After a general anesthetic, ask for your baby to be given to you as soon
as you waken. A helper can put your baby to your breast, at least for a
cuddle, even if you are not fully awake. You can learn how to feed her
once you have recovered from the anesthetic. In the meantime you and
she will have had time together, she may even have had a chance to feed,
and your breasts will have been stimulated to start making milk.

If you have given birth to more than one baby, then you can still cuddle and feed, but probably just with one baby at a time. Your partner or helper can share by cuddling the other baby or babies.

If your baby is taken to the intensive or special care nursery, then you can still stimulate your breasts to produce milk soon after delivery. Go see your baby and, if you can, touch or hold her as soon as possible; this will help you and also help your milk supply. Then ask for help in expressing your milk (see pages 89–94 about expression).

Express in the first few hours after birth, and then every three hours or so, regularly, until you can feed your baby. Ask to hold her, or at least touch and stroke her, before you express, as this will help your milk to flow.

Remember that even if your baby does not feed for some time after birth, but needs intravenous fluids or tube feeding, she will still be able to feed from your breasts when she is well enough. The important thing is to keep your breasts stimulated, so that when she can feed, you have plenty of milk. If you have trouble doing this, try not to worry. Once she is well enough to feed from your breasts, her feeding will soon stimulate your milk (see pages 102–104 for more information on babies who need special care).

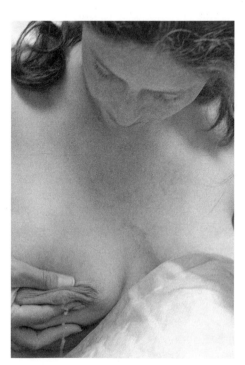

If for any reason your baby cannot breastfeed, start to express your milk so that your baby can still have it.

Before you start any breastfeed, remember that like any meal, you first need to prepare it. The more careful the preparation, the better the food. Here is a simple way of relaxing.

> Before you begin to feed, take three quiet, slow breaths, focusing your full attention on the sensation of simply breathing in and breathing out.
>
> Listen to the sound of the air as it passes down the back of your throat.
>
> Feel your chest and abdomen expand the way a round balloon fills, as the air enters and fills your body, bringing with it the calm you need.
>
> Imagine your breath is your best friend, one who is always there for you, always ready to soothe you when you are tired or stressed.

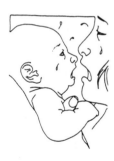

It is especially important to calm yourself before you try to help your baby if she is crying or upset. It takes only a few seconds. Then, when you are calm, take the time to comfort her. If you cannot calm her, have someone else take her and comfort her. Do this before you try to put her to your breast. It really makes a difference.

To get breastfeeding right, you first need to understand three important aspects:

1. *The way you and your baby are positioned during feeding*

2. *How your body works to produce and release milk*

3. *How the composition of your milk changes in the course of a single feed*

These points are described in detail in the next sections.

Position Matters

☆ *Good positioning means getting yourself and your baby into comfortable, effective body positions.* When you learn to drive a car, you need to be sitting comfortably in the driver's seat, hands on the wheel and feet on the pedals. You *could* reach the pedals and the wheel by stretching your legs and arms if the seat was too far back from the pedals and wheel or tilted back too far. But it would not be comfortable, effective, or safe, and you would be bound to run into problems.

Or imagine you are learning to type. It's much easier to sit in a good position, so that your body and arms are comfortable. If you are well positioned on a comfortable chair, you will get less tired while typing, and you'll be more accurate too.

Learning to breastfeed is just the same. You may be able to do it if one or both of you is in an awkward position, but it is a recipe for problems in the long run. It's worth the effort to get positioned correctly right from the beginning.

Remember that mothers and babies, everywhere, always have to *learn* to breastfeed. Like driving a car, typing, or any other skill, some of us learn faster than others. And with breastfeeding there are two of you learning together!

Remember too that for breastfeeding to work well, it does not matter what size your baby is or what shape your nipples are. *Babies don't nipple feed; they breastfeed.*

It doesn't matter how small or big your breasts or nipples are. They are the right size. You can still breastfeed well if you have inverted nipples, although you will need skilled help at first (see pages 95–97).

The information given here is especially for mothers of new babies. Most women find that after they and their babies learn about breastfeeding, they can do it in almost any position, anywhere, at any time. For some it comes easily, straightaway. But at first, for many women, it requires concentration, patience, and practice while learning.

Getting Positioning Right

You need to think about three things as you learn to get positioning right. These are:

1. **Your posture:** Whatever posture you are in, whether you are sitting up or lying down, ask yourself when you start, Am I really comfortable? It is hard to feed your baby well if your back, neck, or shoulder is strained, your arm tired, or your bottom hurts.

2. **How you hold your baby:** Ask yourself, Am I holding my baby's body close enough to me? Can he reach my breast comfortably, without having to make an effort?

3. **How your baby takes your breast:** Ask yourself, Is he able to take a good mouthful of my breast without having to pull at my nipple?

A NOTE TO HELPERS If you are helping, ask yourself, Where am I in relation to this mother and her baby? If you are not in a comfortable position yourself, you may not be able to give the time it takes to help her. Your discomfort may distract you, and she may pick up on your feelings and be ill at ease.

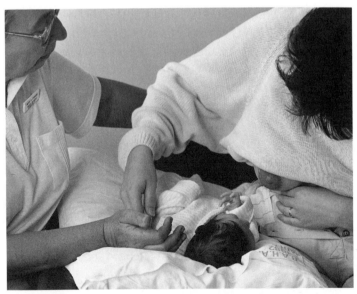

Your helper must be sitting in a comfortable position alongside you to give you the greatest assistance.

Your Posture

From the very first feed, try not to forget *yourself* in the excitement of putting your baby to your breast. It's still the same as in pregnancy and birth. Whatever you do affects your baby—and the better you look after yourself, the happier your baby will be.

Your body needs to be in a posture where you can hold your baby's body tucked in close to you, and in which your breast does not pull away from her mouth as she feeds.

This means that if you are sitting, you need to be upright, not leaning backward. Look at the pictures here: look at how the woman's breast shape and the direction of her nipple change as she sits upright,

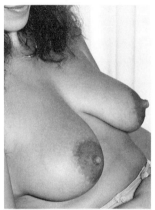
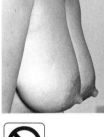
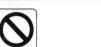

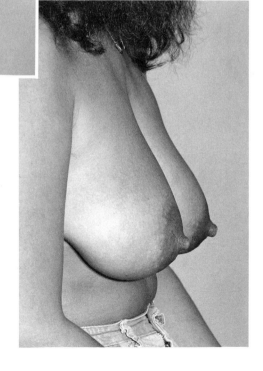

The way you sit (or lie) affects the angle of your breasts and therefore the amount of breast your baby can take.

In the first photograph above (left) the woman is leaning back and her nipple points upward.

In the photograph above (right) she leans too far forward and her nipple points downward.

In this photograph, she is sitting up with her back straight and her breast is in a good position for the baby to take.

as compared to leaning back in the chair. Your baby will not be able to get as good a mouthful of your breast if you lean back. Your breast should never be stretched or pulled in the process of feeding.

Start by getting yourself into a body position in which you feel comfortable. There are a variety of possible positions: you and your baby will work out the ones that are good for both of you. You will probably use different positions at different times. A few suggestions are

- **Try sitting in a straight-backed chair if you have one.** This chair should allow your feet to be flat on the floor and your lap flat or your knees just slightly higher than your lap. See the photo at the bottom of the next page.

  Your legs should not come up markedly toward your chest, as they would in a very low chair. And your thighs should not slope down toward the floor, as they would if the chair was too high. If you have a chair that is too high for you, then use a footstool or books to raise your legs, or tuck your feet up on the crossbar of the chair if it has one. You may also need a pillow on your lap to bring the baby up closer to your breast.

- **If you do not have a simple straight-backed chair, you can use an armchair or sofa.** But be sure to tuck pillows down behind your back—lower back, upper back, and shoulders, as in the picture here—to support you in an upright position. Many big chairs are deep, and you will need several pillows, cushions, folded blankets, or rugs tucked around you before your back will be straight and your feet flat on the floor.

- **Try sitting on the edge of your bed.** You will have nothing behind your back for support, but you can easily lean slightly forward with your feet on the floor. Use a footstool or books under your feet if the bed is too high. If you are using a hospital bed, you may need to rest your feet on a chair. Put some pillows on your lap to support both your baby and your arms until you get used to this position.

  Note: Be especially careful if you choose to feed sitting up in bed. It can be done, but it is more difficult to get truly upright when your legs are stretched out in front of you or tucked up crosslegged. Tuck pillows behind your back. If you have to be in bed, it is probably better to feed lying down.

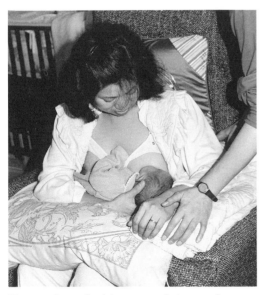

You can breastfeed in an armchair or soft couch—BUT first tuck pillows or cushions down behind your back to support yourself upright. Placing another pillow or two on your lap, so that your baby is supported at the height of your breast takes strain off your shoulders and back.

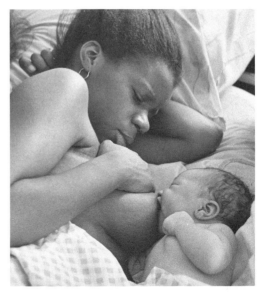

Lying on your side is also a good way to feed. It may be the only comfortable position for a few days if you have had a cesarean or have a spinal headache and need to remain lying down.

This woman is feeding from the upper breast. To do this she has placed her baby on a thick, firm cushion which supports her body completely and frees her mother's arms.

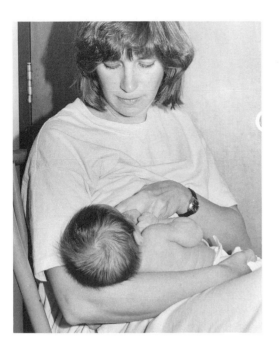

This woman is sitting upright and supporting her baby at the height of her breast (by crossing one knee over the other and resting her forearm her thigh). What is wrong with this picture?

She has placed the baby's head in the crook of her arm, as if she were bottle feeding (which means that to feed, her baby must pull her breast to the side). Instead, she needs to place the baby a few inches down her forearm.

• **You can also lie on your side.** This is especially good if you have just given birth and are in bed, have a sore bottom, or have had a cesarean. You can lie anywhere comfortable: your bed, a long sofa, or the floor.

For this, you will probably need help with the first few feeds, both to lie down comfortably and to position your baby. Once you are lying down, you can really use only one arm to help yourself with feeding, as you will lie on or support your weight with the other, so you need someone to put the baby exactly where you want him.

Lying on your side you can choose to feed from either your lower breast (the one closest to the surface you are lying on) or your upper breast. To use the upper breast, you will need to support yourself slightly up on your elbow and turn your upper body so you are leaning over your baby, or let your breast fall into her mouth. Or place your baby up on pillows so that she is level with your breast. Look at the picture here to see how to do it. Note especially the support from pillows, cushions, and blankets that is needed to keep you and your baby close together when you are lying down.

You may wish to lie with your head and back supported a bit higher than your hips and legs are, like the woman in the picture here. If you are in a hospital bed, you can ask someone to raise the back of the bed so your upper body is at a slight angle. At home some big cushions or pillows would have the same effect.

• **You don't need a chair, sofa, or bed.** You can sit on the floor with your back straight, your legs crossed (as in the photograph on page 43) or in the tailor position (where you sit with your knees open and your feet together). You can put pillows in the hollow between your knees. It is easier if you have a wall behind you. Do keep your back straight.

Experiment with different postures, and try them out to see how they feel for you before you put your baby to your breast. When you read our descriptions in the next section of the positions your baby should be in, you will see why your own posture matters so much.

Lying on your side can be an easy way to
breastfeed and nap at the same time once you
and your baby have learned how to do it.

To breastfeed well in this position, remember
to tuck your baby close in to your body (her
entire body against yours) and have her head
level with your breast so that she does not
have to reach for or pull on it.

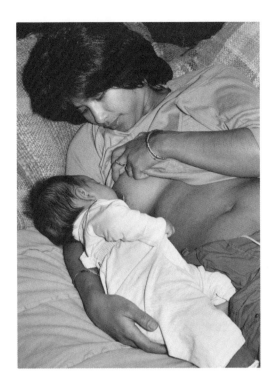

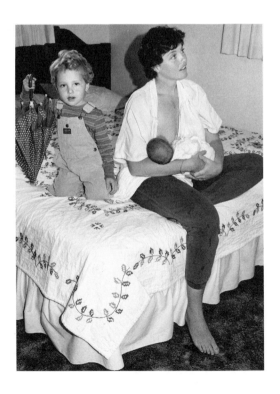

You can sit on the edge of the bed to feed, but
make sure at least one foot is flat on the
floor (putting something under your feet to
raise them if you need to). Also remember to
keep your back straight and have your baby's
head at the height of your breast.

This woman's breasts are low; her baby can
lie on her arm and her arm can rest on her thigh
without her having to bend her back.

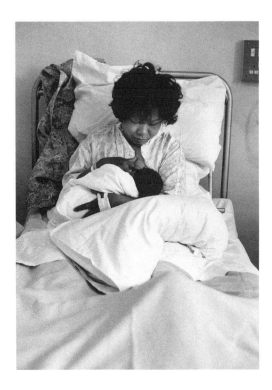

Breastfeeding while sitting up in bed is difficult. If you do this, then have something firm behind to support you sitting upright.

This mother's breasts are high. She needs a pillow under the baby to bring the baby to the right height, so that she does not need to carry the baby's weight in her arms, shoulders, and back.

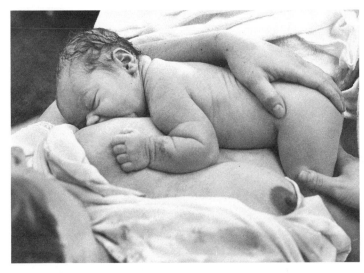

If necessary, you can feed your baby while lying on your back. This is not always easy— it may be difficult for the baby to take enough of your breast and may not stimulate your milk supply enough. It is not recommended for most women.

This mother must temporarily lie on her back to feed, so she drapes her newborn baby's body over hers, and makes sure that the baby takes not only the nipple but a lot of breast tissue in his mouth.

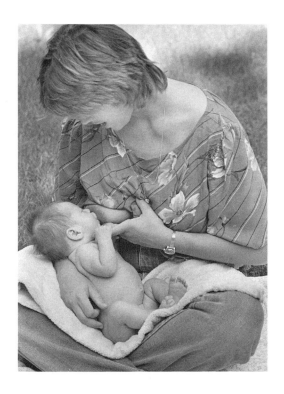

Once you are confident and breastfeeding is going well, then you can breastfeed anywhere and in a variety of positions that work well for you and your baby.

This position would be very difficult for a newborn. The baby, who is four weeks old, is well supported (with his head at the level of his mother's breast and his body resting on a folded towel in her lap) but his body is not facing his mother's, nor is it tucked in close, so he must turn his head to feed.

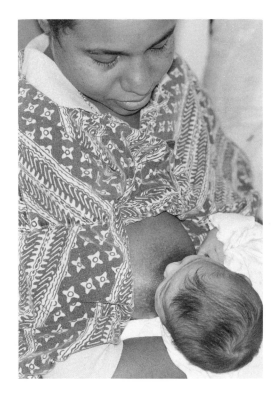

This mother has turned her five-day-old baby's body toward hers and tucked her in close before starting to feed. The baby's head rests on her forearm (not in the crook of her elbow), and she supports her baby's lower back and bottom with her hand.

In summary, the important principles of your posture to get right are:

1. **Make yourself comfortable.** Your body needs to be well supported, so you can hold your baby close to your breast for half an hour or more without your arms getting too tired. If you are comfortable and well-supported you will not have to use any extra effort to hold your baby, and you will not get back, shoulder, or neck tension.

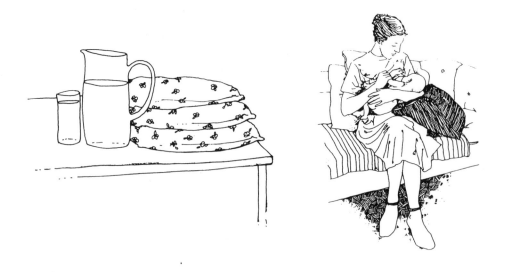

2. **Make sure you are not leaning back**—so that your breasts are not pulled away from your baby and out of his mouth while he tries to feed—or hunched over.

3. **Use props for support.** Have as many pillows, cushions, or soft, firm supports (such as folded rugs or blankets as well as whatever you may need to support your feet) as you need to support both you and your baby.

4. **Remember to have a glass of water** or other beverage within your reach so you can drink something while breastfeeding, if you are thirsty.

5. **While getting yourself ready**, you may need to put the baby down beside you or have someone else hold the baby until you are ready to have him brought to you.

Two important things to avoid:

- *Do not* be tempted to sit leaning back in bed, or in a chair that is designed for lounging, without proper support behind your back.

- *Do not* be tempted to start feeding until you are comfortable and ready.

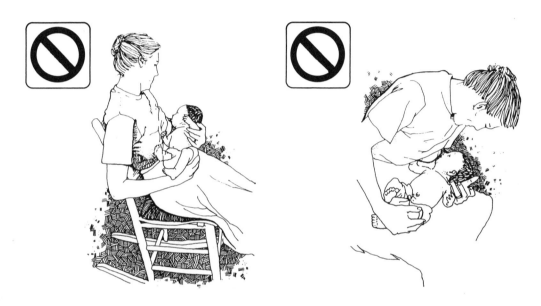

Once you and your baby have got breastfeeding right, you will get so used to feeding that you'll do it along with all your ordinary activities—while you are on the phone, eating your dinner, or working at your desk. You'll have a spare hand for reading, cuddling your older child, or holding a cup. At the start, though, learn what is most comfortable for you.

How You Hold Your Baby

Once you are comfortable, you need to hold your baby in a good position for her to be able to feed. *She needs to be comfortable, well supported, and not straining to get at your breast.*

You may find, at first, that it is easier for you to hold your baby with one arm or the other, depending on whether you are right-handed or left-handed. With practice, it will get easier with the other arm.

If you have twins, practice feeding just one baby at a time at first. When you are good at it, you can try both at once.

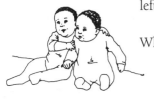

- **Hold your baby tucked in very close to your body, with her body turned in toward yours, so she is lying on her side.** She should not have to turn her head to reach your breast. Her front should be tucked in close to your body, secure but not tight.

There are no rules about which of your hands should be used for what. The important things are:

1. *Your baby should feel secure and supported.*

2. *She must have good, easy access to your breast.*

Look at the pictures in this section. Note how the women are holding their babies. Even though the babies are in similar positions close to their mothers, the women are holding them differently. *Work out what is best for you and your baby.*

- **Her whole body, especially from her head to her bottom, should be well supported.** Use your hands and arms and possibly pillows too to support her if you are sitting up. If you are lying down, she will be lying on her side on the bed or floor, on pillows or on your arm.

- **She needs to be held so that her mouth will be at the same level as your nipple when she feeds.** She should not have to pull down or away from your breast once she is on your breast. This means that she should not be held above the level of your nipple. If anything, she should be held *just below* your nipple as you prepare to bring her to your breast.

- **Her head, neck, and back should be in almost a straight line.** Her head should not be tilted down. She will not be able to swallow in that position. If anything, her head should be tilted *slightly* backward, so her chin presses into your breast.

It is important that a young baby's body and head are in a straight line during feeding. The head must be at the level of the mother's breast, but the body can slope downward, as long as it does not cause the baby to pull down on the breast.

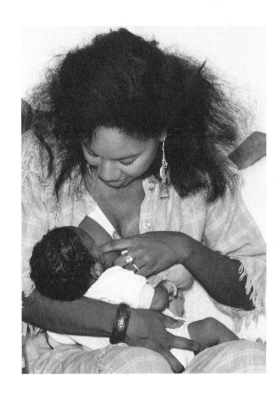

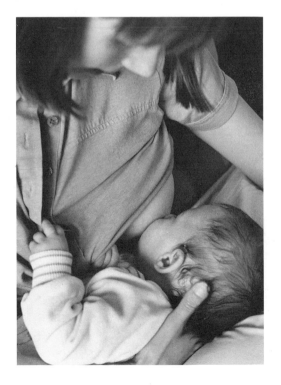

This is good positioning. Here a mother supports her baby's neck and shoulders in her hand, with her thumb and fingers resting on the back of his head. Notice how the baby's chin is neither tilted up nor dropped back.

Note: Good positioning for your baby never requires her to turn her head to take your breast when she is young. Whatever position you and she are in, cradle her close to you, with her mouth in front of and just below your nipple. Look carefully at the pictures in this book, and look at how well supported the babies are, and how close they are to their mothers' bodies.

A special tip on your clothing: Wearing comfortable clothing helps in getting positioning right. If you have to fuss with tight or uncomfortable clothes, it will get in the way of you and your baby. Try to wear clothes that are comfortable and in which you can feed discreetly if you are outside your home. A big shawl or scarf can be useful here. A loose top that can be pulled up is often more discreet and comfortable than a blouse that buttons down the front.

 In summary, the important points to remember about how you hold your baby are that your baby:

1. *Is held close to you*

2. *Is well supported*

3. *Is facing you*

4. *Has her mouth just below your nipple as you prepare to feed*

5. *Has her head, neck, and back all in a straight line*

6. *Make sure her arms and hands do not get in the way as she goes on to feed*

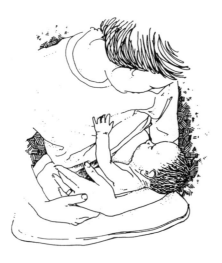
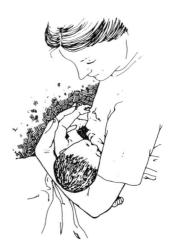

The important things to avoid are as follows:

- *Do not* lie your baby on her back. She would have to turn her head to find your breast.

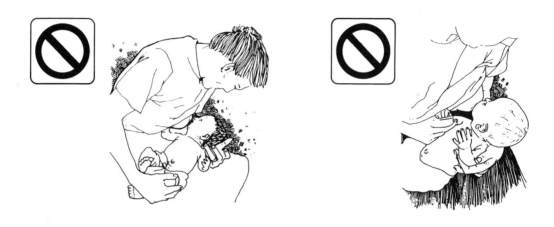

- *Do not* hold her so that her mouth is above or well below your nipple.

- *Do not* let her chin push down toward her chest.

- *Do not* bring your breast to the baby, bring your baby to the breast.

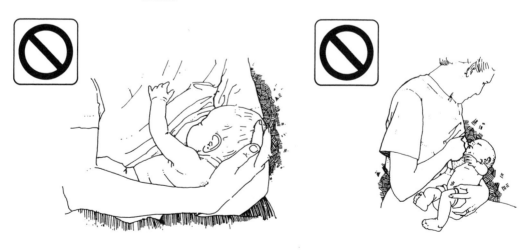

A Note on Supporting Your Breast

 Once you and your baby are confident with breastfeeding, you may not need to support your breast. But in the early days it can often help.

Breast support may be necessary only while you are putting your baby onto your breast. Once she is on and suckling, some women will not require this support.

You can use either hand, under either breast. Use whichever hand is not supporting your baby. Cup your hand underneath your breast, with four fingers underneath and your thumb resting lightly on top.

Remember, you are *supporting* it, not holding it tightly. Just feel the weight of your breast in your hand. Look carefully at the picture here of how to do this.

Your hand is simply supporting your breast to make it a bit firmer as your baby goes on, and to lift it slightly so your baby is not supporting its weight with his chin. It is not intended to squeeze your breast into a different shape; that will not help, and may pull the breast partly out of your baby's mouth. Be especially careful not to let your thumb press into your breast. You may be able to remove your hand once your baby is feeding well.

If you have small breasts, you may not need to support them at all.

If you have large breasts, you may need to support them throughout the whole feed.

This woman, who has large breasts, is using a band of soft material (a long stretch of broad bandage or a long woven belt would do) tied around her neck, looped under her breast. It is tied tight enough to give good support to her breast, but not tight enough to distort the shape of the part of the breast and the nipple offered to her baby. It can be slipped off the first breast and looped under the second breast when necessary.

If you are out and about when feeding, then carry this band with you. It would be best to wear a front-fastening blouse; just slip the band over your head and around your breast, and feed as normal.

Alternatively, use your hand under your breast throughout the feed, as the woman in this picture is doing.

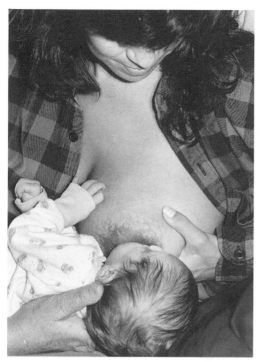

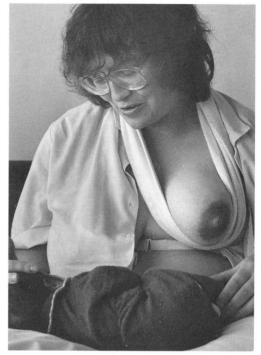

This baby's shoulders and head are well supported with the opposite hand, so the mother's other hand is free to support her breast. Note how she keeps her thumb well back from the areola and does not press it down on the breast.

This woman has large, soft breasts. She is using a band of soft material (an elasticized fabric) around her neck and under her breast to give it support and better shape for the baby to suckle. This way both of her hands are free to support her newborn and help him take her breast.

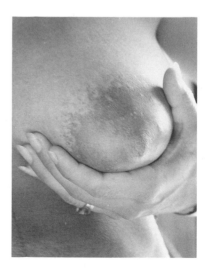

If you need to support your breast, place your fingers and palm of the hand underneath and rest your thumb lightly either on top of the breast (but well back from the areola) or back toward your armpit. This way you are less likely to distort the shape of the breast as the baby feeds.

How Your Baby Takes Your Breast

 These principles of how your baby takes your breast are the same for all mothers and babies, even if you have inverted nipples or a small or sick baby. It will be more difficult if you have these problems. It will probably take longer and you will need lots of patience, but it can work! (See pages 95–97 if you have inverted nipples, and pages 102–107 if you have a small or sick baby.)

This part will work well only if you have arranged yourself and your baby comfortably and well. If you and he are comfortably together, then you will be able to carry out these steps to encourage him to take your breast.

- **Support your baby well** across his shoulder and the base of his head. You can do this in either of two ways:

  a. Cradle him on the inside of your forearm, on the same side on which he is feeding. You will support his shoulders and neck on your arm just below your elbow.

  b. Support him with the arm on the opposite side from the breast he is feeding from. Cradle his shoulders, his neck, and the base of his head lightly on your hand. This is for support only. Do not put pressure on his head. His back should rest on the inside of your forearm.

- **Hold his head gently.**

- **Brush your baby's lips lightly against your nipple**, to give him a sense of what to take in his mouth. If he is well positioned, he should already be right by your nipple.

- **Wait until his mouth is wide open before letting him take your breast in his mouth.** He has a reflex to do this; you simply need to encourage this reflex.

  When his mouth is opening wide, *and not until* it is opening like a yawn, quickly move his head onto your breast so he can take a good, deep mouthful. (This may take practice to get the timing right. If you wait too long, he will have begun to close his mouth by the time you bring him onto the breast.)

  You may have to work with this for a few minutes before he gapes his mouth open widely enough to take in enough of your breast. Don't worry about this. Some babies are sleepy. Some

A newborn baby's head is very sensitive and needs to be held gently, especially if the baby has had a difficult passage at birth.

This mother places the palm of her hand on her baby's upper back and shoulders, leaving her fingers free to bring the baby on to her breast.

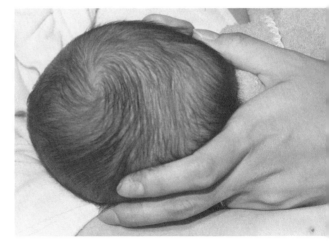

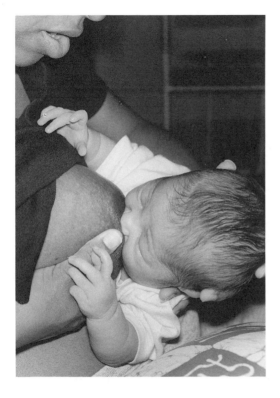

This mother is sitting upright and using the opposite arm to hold her baby so that her baby's nose is at the level of her nipple.

Notice how she gently cradles the baby's head with her fingers, which gives her just enough control to make sure the baby is well on the breast. By resting this arm on a pillow she avoids strain to her back and shoulders.

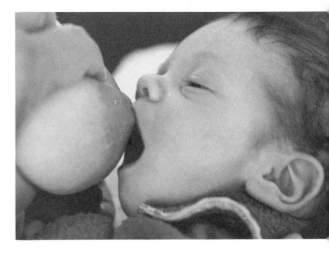

Look at this baby's wide gape and how his nostrils are at the level of the nipple. This is the correct position for the baby going on the breast, since it is actually the baby's lower jaw, pressed in against the breast, that does the work.

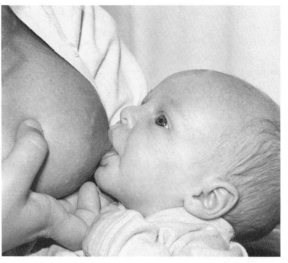

This baby is not well on the breast. He is nipple feeding, not breastfeeding. If he were allowed to continue to do this, his mother would become very sore.

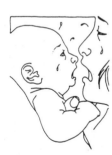

are not too hungry. *All babies have to learn to feed well.* Calmly repeat the action of lightly brushing his lips against your nipple until he responds by opening his mouth wide.

If he or you become frustrated or cry, then stop. Breathe. Calm down. Calm him. Try again. It does not matter if feeding takes a long time in the early days; you will both become better as you practice. If you are both crying or if you are tense, it helps to have someone else calm the baby and calm you. Ask for a back rub or neck massage or cup of tea or whatever will make you feel better.

- **Make sure he takes a large mouthful of your breast, not just your nipple.** To do this, he needs to use his whole bottom jaw and tongue. Think about where the baby's bottom lip, rather than his top lip, makes contact with your breast. (It is his lower jaw that does the work in extracting your milk.) Your nipple will then end up right at the back of his mouth, where it cannot be damaged by suction or friction.

  Look at the diagram and photograph here to see where your nipple should be. Look too at how your baby's tongue should lie right over his gum, covering it. In this position his tongue and bottom jaw will move rhythmically up and down against your breast to get the milk. His tongue will lie over his bottom gum throughout the feed; it will not move in and out. In fact, you (or someone guiding you) may see his tongue if you just tip back the edge of his lower lip while he is feeding well (but be careful not to disturb him if you do this).

The photograph of the baby with her tongue on her lower gum shows you where the tongue is when feeding well.

The mouthful of breast that he takes in should be all the way around and behind your nipple, and include some of the dark area around your nipple (the areola). Some women with small areolas find that the baby takes it all in; some women with large areolas still can see quite a lot of it.

If you can still see some areola, more of it should show beyond your baby's top lip than beyond his bottom lip. *It will be hard for you to see this, because it is impossible to see looking down on yourself.*

This baby has just come off the breast. You can still see her tongue, which is thrust forward during breastfeeding and completely covers her lower gum.

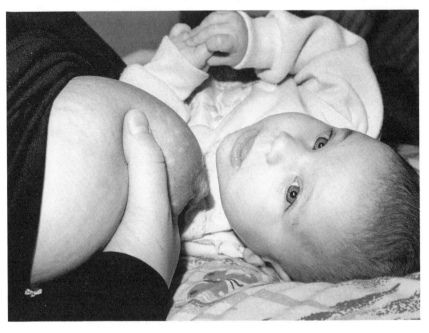

You cannot easily see under your own breast. You can ask a helper what your baby and breast look like when he is feeding, or sit beside a mirror to see for yourself. The picture on page 60 shows what it should look like.

Remember that breastfed babies *take* the breast: it is not like bottle feeding, where babies are *given* the teat or bottle nipple.

(In some countries, such as the United States, the word *nipple* is used for the rubber or plastic tip of the bottle on which the baby sucks. In this book we use the word *nipple* only to describe the nipple on a woman's breast; this is sensitive, stretchy, and responsive. Rubber or plastic objects are not. We use the word *teat* throughout this book to describe the rubber or plastic tip of the bottle.)

- **Relax and let the feed happen.** If for any reason you feel your baby is not well positioned, especially if it is painful for you, stop the feed. Take him off your breast gently by breaking the suction; you can do this by slipping a finger in his mouth. (It is best to do this with short fingernails.) Take a few slow breaths to calm yourself. Then calm him and start again.

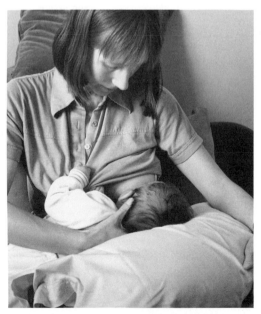

Once your baby is feeding well, there is
nothing else you need to do. You can relax and
enjoy it.

This three-month-old baby is well supported, with a hand behind her shoulders and fingers cradling her head. Her body rests on her mother's lap.

If this were a young infant, then her body would need to be turned on its side and tucked in close. This detail is not so important for an older infant, who can easily turn from the waist.

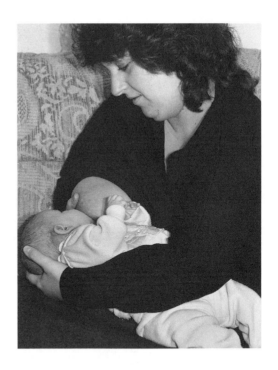

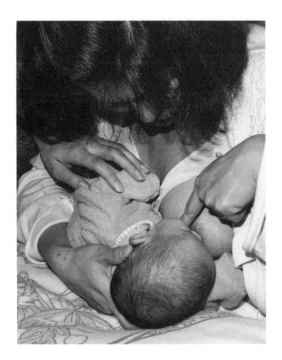

Here is how to break suction gently, if you need to take the baby off your breast.

Place your finger in her mouth, press down on your breast tissue (which breaks the suction), and draw your nipple out as you take her off.

What to Do if Breastfeeding Hurts

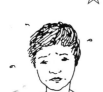

Breastfeeding should not hurt, other than a brief pain during the first few sucks of each feed, in the first few days (or for the first day or two after you have begun working on a problem). If it hurts, then usually the positioning is not right. Stop feeding; gently take your baby off your breast. Take a few calming breaths and try again.

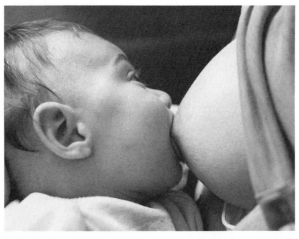

This baby is not well positioned. Can you see how this positioning may not permit the baby to get enough milk (and therefore not stimulate enough milk to be produced for the next feed) and would be likely to result in sore nipples or worse?

Note how she seems to be pulling down and off the breast. There is also a gap between her chin and the breast and her nose is not resting against the breast.

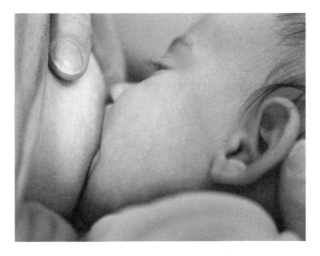

Here this same baby is positioned just right on the opposite breast. She is now tucked in close to the breast, her mouth open wide, and her chin against the underside of the breast. She has taken in a good mouthful and is feeding well.

Because nipple pain and damage is usually caused by positioning problems, there is no need to use any of the over-the-counter or prescription creams, sprays, and lotions that may be recommended to you, or that you may see in drug or chemist shops. These can actually cause nipple damage by interfering with the normal balance of organisms on the skin. Nor do you need to prepare your nipples in pregnancy (by using methods that supposedly toughen and prevent them from getting sore or cracked), or prepare them by washing them before you feed. If the positioning is right, then nothing else is needed. You or a helper can look for these signs to see if your baby is feeding well:

1. Your baby should have gaped his mouth widely enough and be tucked in close enough that he should have taken a large mouthful of breast.

2. Your baby's upper lip should be pressed against the breast, not pinching in at the base of the nipple.

3. His nose should not dig into your breast; if it does he is not well positioned. *There should be no need for you to hold your breast away from his nose to let him breathe.* You should see his top lip splayed back and up and a small gap between that and his splayed nostrils. Tuck his body in closer to you, if necessary, to widen the gap a little between his nose and your breast.

4. His bottom lip should be turned back against your breast, and his bottom jaw should be firmly pressing into the underside of your breast.

   This is hard for you to see, but you should be able to feel the sensation from the tip of the tongue and the jaw moving together at a point that is well onto your breast, *not* up close to your nipple.

   Do not try to look at this part in too much detail, as moving your baby or your breast to have a look will disturb your baby. Instead, shut your eyes and feel the sensation of his tongue and jaws. Remember that it should not hurt at all.

5. Your baby will take a few quick sucks, and then start to suck strongly, deeply, and rhythmically. You will notice that he will have a pattern of sucking a few times and then pausing, sucking again a few times and then pausing again.

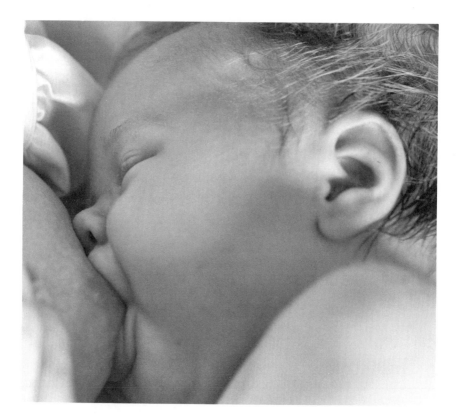

When breastfeeding is going well, the mother's nipple is never damaged because it is so far back in the baby's mouth that there is no friction against it. (It is friction that causes both soreness and damage to the nipple.) This is why breastfeeding should not hurt.

In this photograph, and the accompanying drawing and diagram, you can see what is going on inside your baby's mouth when breastfeeding is going well.

Notice that when the baby is well on the breast her lower lip is pressed down flat against her chin and she has taken not only the nipple but also a large amount of breast tissue into her mouth, forming them into a teat with her tongue.

The baby's nose is against the breast but not pressing in. You can see how the nostrils in this drawing flare to the side, which makes it possible for her nose to be right against your breast and for her still to be able to breathe. Look at your baby and see how her nostrils are designed so that she can breathe comfortably while breastfeeding.

In the diagram, see how your baby's tongue should completely cover her lower gum (or teeth) and protect your nipple, which lies safely in the back of the baby's mouth where it cannot be damaged.

You can see very little of this mother's large areola, because most of it is in the baby's mouth. Look at how the nipple plus breast tissue together are pulled into the shape of a teat.

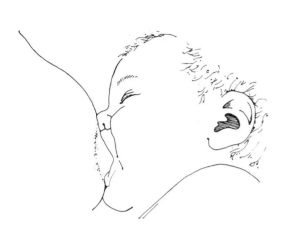
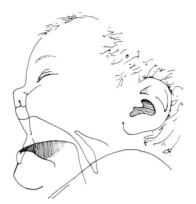

KEY:

1—nipple

2—areola and breast tissue, with underlying
    milk ducts

3—baby's tongue

4—breast

5—baby's throat

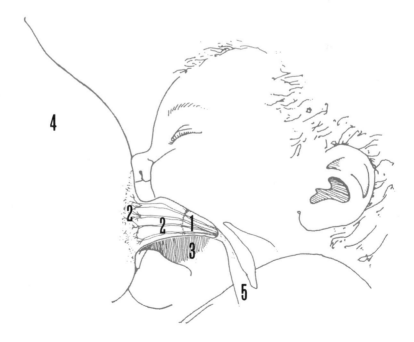

He will do this throughout the feed. He will vary the strength of his sucks every now and then, but mostly they should be regular, deep, and strong.

As the feed goes on, he will pause for longer periods, and the bouts of sucking will get shorter. Do not be tempted to take him off the breast at this point. He needs to continue feeding. This is explained on page 77.

6. Your baby will continue to feed peacefully and well until he decides he has had enough. At that time he will let go of your breast. *There is no need for you to take him off. He will show you that he has had enough when that time comes.*

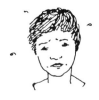

7. Feeding should not hurt you. People mistakenly think that pain is a normal part of breastfeeding. It is not. You may feel an unusual sensation as his sucking stretches your nipple. Some women even feel a quick stab of pain around the nipple just as the baby starts, which passes in a few seconds. That will last only for the first few days.

One sensation you may feel is a strong tingling, like a mild electrical charge, as you release your milk (see page 73). This too is normal, although not something women usually feel in the early days or weeks. It is also normal not to feel any tingling at all; some women do, some don't.

Special tip: Occasionally some babies who are feeding well come off the breast for a few seconds, not long after they have started to feed. Then they soon go back on again. These babies show no signs of distress, and there is no pain for the mothers. We believe that these babies need to come off briefly, either because the milk flow is too fast to cope with, or because they need to burp or pass wind.

Once your baby has taken the first side well, he will want a short rest. He may or may not decide to take the second side (see page 78).

After your baby is finished with one breast, it is a good moment to change his diaper or nappy if necessary. You can then see if he is interested in taking the second side. *Give him the choice.* He may be finished.

The same principles of positioning apply to the second side. Be just as careful, let him come off the breast himself when he has finished.

Some babies cry immediately after a good feed. Hunger can be eliminated as a cause. See pages 137–144 for what to do if this happens.

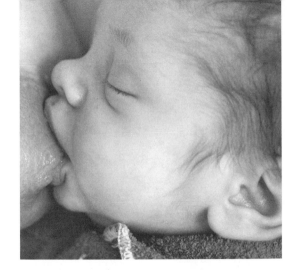

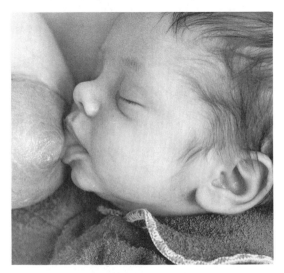

In this series you can see how the baby comes off the breast by herself when she has had enough.

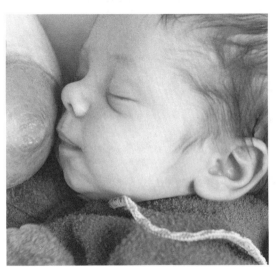

In summary, what is important about how your baby takes your breast is that at each feed your baby should:

1. *Gape his mouth widely.*

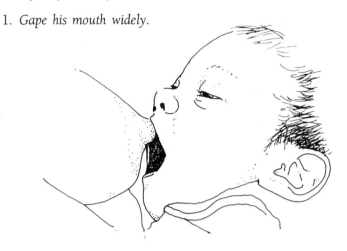

2. *Take a large mouthful of breast.*

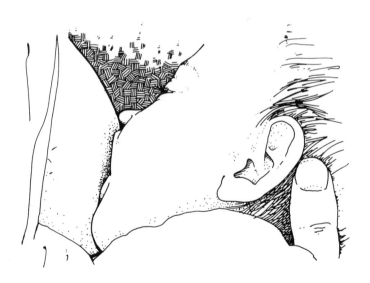

3. *Suck mostly strongly and rhythmically, with pauses between each episode of sucking.*

4. *Have no problem breathing.*

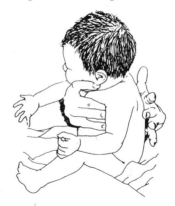

5. *Easily bring up any air bubbles (burp/wind) if you sit him up. Remember to support his head.*

6. *Come off the breast himself when he has finished.*

Remember that feeding should not hurt you at all.

☆ **The important things to avoid are as follows:**

- *Do not* try to put your breast into your baby's mouth. Simply help him take it by moving him to your breast.

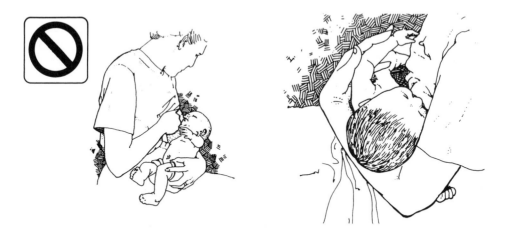

- *Do not* let him feed if it hurts you; take him off and try again.

- *Do not* let him continue to feed if he sucks rapidly and lightly *all the time*. Take him off and try again.

- *Do not* continue to feed if he seems distressed. Calm yourself, calm him, and try again.

One Mother's Experience of Learning to Breastfeed Well: *The First Two Weeks*

With my first child, Colin, I had sore, cracked nipples, and breastfeeding didn't become pleasant for six weeks. That's how long it took for me to learn how to put him on my breast right and for him to know what to do. I didn't realize he was sucking on my nipple and that's why I was sore. Once he was on my breast, I let him stay for half an hour or more or until he fell asleep because he would scream if I took him off. Colin never came off the breast on his own. Sometimes I would hardly get a break between feeds.

Finally I found a breastfeeding support group listed in the phone directory. I called, told them my symptoms, and asked for help. I was able to heal my nipples, even the cracked one, by letting them air after each feed until they were completely dry and by teaching Colin to take much more of the breast in his mouth. For a while I had to pay close attention each time I put him on or he would not get it right. Once we learned to breastfeed correctly, everything was fine. He didn't wean fully until eighteen months, and by that time he was only taking my breast for a few minutes several times a day, for comfort.

I have big nipples, and both my babies have had small mouths. Colin was born with the habit of sucking his bottom lip and not opening his mouth very wide to feed. I had to teach him how to take my breast. And I have had to do the same with Devi, my daughter.

Devi sucked strongly from the first feed, and she has always opened her mouth wide. She seemed to take my breast well until my milk came in fully at forty-eight hours. I think my breast was really stimulated to produce because she sucked so strongly. I suddenly be-

came very full and that, combined with the size of my nipples and the fact that they didn't stand erect, prevented her from getting my breast into her mouth. She began to scream at each feed, to shake her head when I put her on, to spit out the nipple, and to refuse the breast. It was a struggle for a few days.

I began to apply warmth to my breasts between feeds, using a heating pad or standing under a warm shower. This made me feel more comfortable, took down some of the swelling, and softened my breast tissue, making it easier for Devi to take my breast. My husband bought a hand pump for me, and I expressed as much milk as I felt comfortable with before each feed. I would drop some milk directly into her mouth when it was open from crying; and as soon as she'd tasted it, I'd put her on while she was still crying and her mouth was open. She would suck two or three times, get upset, pull off, and start crying again. The third and fourth days after her birth were the hardest. At first I was very upset, and I was afraid of repeating what had happened with Colin.

I tried to keep myself calm, but it was hard for those two days. She seemed so hungry and yet so upset (as upset as I was)! Once, during the night, my husband gave her a bottle of my expressed milk, and the next afternoon I fed her another bottle to make sure she would not lose weight. Then I called my midwife; she stayed on the phone, talking me through a whole feed. Then she suggested I send my husband to get me a beer so I would relax—that helped too.

My husband is very helpful. He is taking off almost a month of vacation time and unpaid leave from his job to be home with us, to take care of Colin, who is twenty-three months, and to run the house. During the hardest days he gave me back rubs whenever I wanted, even in the middle of the night.

For the entire first week we kept the answering machine on, and I talked on the phone only a little each day, and never when I was feeding Devi. Colin is very active and our house is very small, a three-room cottage with a tiny yard, but we tried to keep it quiet and played soft music. That helped all of us. We also tried to keep visitors to a minimum. We put a sign on our door and told our friends and relatives who dropped by or called that we would love for them to bring us meals but that we probably couldn't spend time with them. Most days

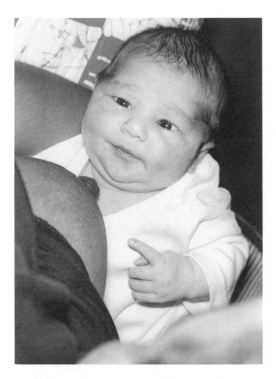

Here, two-day-old Devi is still learning how to take her mother's breast, which is already quite large and firm and has a large nipple that does not stand erect. Like her brother before her, Devi has a small mouth compared to the size of her mother's nipple and breast.

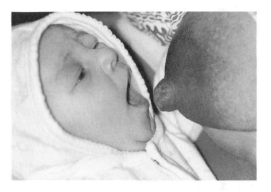

Breastfeeding in situations like this takes time, and practice, and a great deal of patience in the first days, as both mother and baby must learn to get it right.

Lawan first had to teach Devi to open her mouth wide before she could have the breast. This was frustrating for Devi for several days, until she learned.

A few babies can be put on the breast when they are crying, while their mouth is open wide. But, as with most babies, this did not work for Devi. She would cry so hard that she didn't notice when the breast was in her mouth. So Lawan first had to calm her and then coax her to open her mouth. Dripping a little breast milk into her mouth when she first began to cry helped.

someone has brought food, and that has been wonderful, allowing us to spend all our time with Colin and Devi.

By the time Devi was thirteen days, I had finally taught her to take my breast well. For a few days, each time I breastfed I encouraged her by talking to her and gently rocking her. I had learned to hold her whole body very close to me and to keep her wrapped because she prefers being swaddled to having her arms and legs free. I had to feed in a sitting position, making sure my back was straight up and down, to make it work. Feeding times got easier and better each day. She fed well once on the breast and came off on her own when she was done. She'd look at me much of the time she fed. We were really lucky; she already slept five hours at a stretch each night.

Devi cried at the breast and fought feeding only in the middle of the night. I think she was very hungry then and became frustrated more easily. She sometimes took ten or fifteen minutes to get going at that feed; but I didn't give her any choice but to take my breast and even-

tually she did! At that point I hadn't needed to express milk in three days; my nipples weren't cracked; and if Devi didn't go on correctly and sucked on the nipple, I immediately took her off and tried again. Even when everything was right, there was sometimes mild soreness during her first few sucks; but after that there was no pain or soreness. I was beginning to really enjoy it!

For the first three weeks I could only breastfeed sitting upright. After that, Devi learned to feed while I was lying on my side, as long as she was not too hungry. When she was four weeks I could nurse sitting or lying anywhere. When Devi was five weeks I began expressing milk regularly so that my husband could give her a bottle of breastmilk each day, which allowed me to have some free time. I find this especially helpful if we are in the car and she gets hungry.

Devi is now six weeks and knows how to go on the breast. She feeds wells and sleeps five or six hours at a stretch each night. She's an alert, peaceful baby. Breastfeeding is great.

Here, ten days after birth, Devi is feeding well. Lawan still has to be careful at each feed, making sure both she and Devi are in good, comfortable positions and that Devi's head is at the level of her breast and her nose at the level of Lawan's nipple before Lawan puts her on.

In this photograph you can see a bit of Devi's right arm, which Lawan has been careful to place underneath her breast so that it does not get in the way and prevent her from tucking Devi in close to her body. Lawan has a pillow supporting her own forearm, upon which Devi's head rests. She uses another pillow to support Devi's lower body.

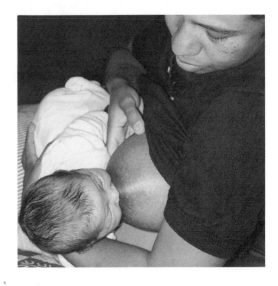

A Note for Helpers

 If you are helping a mother to breastfeed, then take the time to think about your own position.

You should be comfortable, so that you can take all the time that you need, without getting uncomfortable or tired.

You will find the positions that suit you best. Two suggested positions are:

- Sitting beside the mother, side by side, facing the same direction (see picture). You should sit on the side opposite the breast the mother is feeding from, on a chair at the same height as her.

- Sitting beside the mother, facing in the opposite direction. Again, you should be on the opposite side from the breast the mother is feeding from, and at the same height as her.

Work with the mother to guide her, rather than doing it for her. She does not need a helper who will only put her baby on her breast and then leave her. The best care is when you suggest to the mother what she can do, and then watch and guide her in getting it right, or put your hands over hers and let her feel what you are doing. Remember to be

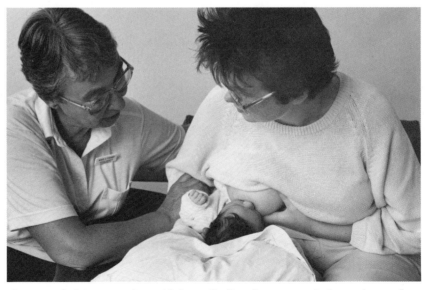

If you are helping a mother with breastfeeding, be sure to sit down close to her. Make sure that your back is comfortable and that you don't have to strain to reach over and assist her.

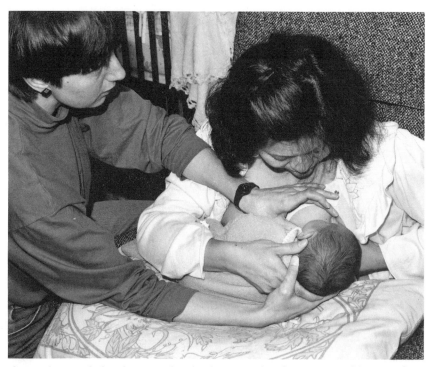

If a mother needs hands-on guidance, place your hands ON TOP of hers so that she can feel how to do it herself. Then watch her do it herself and give her feedback.

patient and reassuring; the most important thing you can give a mother is confidence. A calm, positive manner is as important as skill in positioning the baby.

The pictures here show you how you can guide the mother's hands.

FOR MOTHERS AND HELPERS It is essential that when a mother needs help, the helper has easy access to both her and her breasts. In most countries this is considered quite normal. In the United States some helpers do not work in this way; for fear of legal action, they do not touch women's breasts. *It is unhelpful and unproductive to try to work with a woman while avoiding touching her breasts.* Some women need skilled hands-on care. If you are one of these women, persist in finding someone who will work directly with you, your baby, and your breasts. Or look in the resource section of this book for organizations that may help.

If all else fails, work with a close friend or family member, using this book to guide you.

About Milk Supply and Milk Release

 While you and your baby are working to get breastfeeding right, your body is also working to get the milk supply and composition right.

Milk Supply

Just as in pregnancy your hormones changed to support a growing baby, so after birth your hormones change to make milk.

Your breasts have already been prepared by the pregnancy hormones, and they are already making the essential early milk, or colostrum, for your baby. These hormones also limit the amount made to the small volume your new baby needs at first. As soon as your baby is born, the milk-producing hormone, prolactin, starts to work on your breasts to make a generous milk supply.

Prolactin responds to your baby feeding at your breasts. As your baby feeds, your brain reads the message that your breasts need to make more milk to replace what your baby is taking. It therefore releases prolactin, which gives the signal to your breasts to make more milk. The milk taken from them is simply replaced.

If your baby does not feed well, then the message your breasts will get is that the baby doesn't need much milk, so they will not produce much.

Understanding this helps you to work out:

1. How to build up a good milk supply

2. How to treat milk supply problems if they occur

3. How to build up a good milk supply even if your baby is small or sick and you cannot feed her directly

Make sure that your baby always feeds well, especially in the early days and weeks as your supply becomes established. Limiting your baby's time on the breast, or not getting her well positioned (so that she doesn't get enough milk) will result in your breasts not getting the message to make enough milk.

This balance between the amount your baby needs and the amount

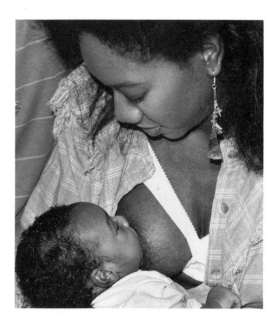

As your baby feeds, your body responds by making more milk to replace what your baby has taken.

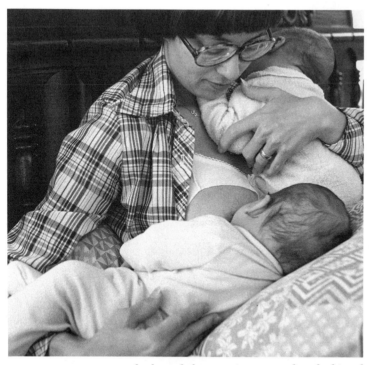

You can produce plenty of milk to feed twins—even triplets. But in the early days it is easier to feed one baby at a time, even though this takes a lot longer. When you become more confident and your babies know how to take the breast, then you can try feeding both babies at once.

your breasts make is so finely tuned that if you have twins, your body will make enough milk for two. All you need to do is help both babies to breastfeed well. Some women have even breastfed triplets (though this is difficult, and you need lots of help).

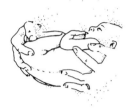

If you cannot feed your baby for a time, then make sure your breasts still get the signal to make milk by removing the milk that is there. If she is in a special care or intensive care unit, if you are so ill you cannot breastfeed, or if you are separated for any other reason, then express your milk regularly (see pages 89–94); or ask for help if you are ill. This is especially important in the first week or two after birth. Do not worry if you do not have much of a supply. You can build up your supply when you and the baby are home.

Milk Release

After producing milk, your breasts need to release it. Milk comes out as a result of a combination of:

1. The letdown reflex and

2. Your baby feeding well

When you feed your baby, or sometimes even if you just think about your baby or hear her cry, your breasts will let down the milk. This means that the small muscles around the areas where milk is stored in your breasts contract and squeeze the milk out.

Some women will feel this letdown like a tingle in their breasts, and others will not feel it at all. Some women find that they feel it more as the baby gets bigger. The surest sign that it is happening is contented swallowing by the baby.

Oxytocin is the hormone responsible for sending the letdown signal to your breasts. This is the same hormone that was responsible for your labor contractions. It is also released when you make love.

You may find that in the early days, your womb contracts whenever you breastfeed. That is oxytocin at work. You will lose more blood around the time of feeding as a result of these contractions, which helps to clear your body of the blood it needs to lose.

With breastfeeding, your womb will also contract down to size more quickly, but it may be painful as it does this. Some women find that these afterbirth contractions, or afterpains, become more painful the more children they have. The feeling will last for only a day or two.

Because oxytocin is also released when you make love, you may find that you release milk at that time. This is normal, but it is useful to have a towel handy so as to avoid a damp bed. It can also help if you feed your baby before making love, to minimize milk release and untimely interruptions by the baby. Because oxytocin is released during both love-making and breastfeeding, some women find that breastfeeding makes them feel sexy. This is quite normal; enjoy it while it lasts.

Sometimes milk is released at times when you do not expect it. Thinking about your baby when you are away from her, or hearing another baby cry can cause milk to let down.

Sometimes women find it hard to release their milk in stressful situations. Oxytocin is not released and the milk will not flow. For this to happen, however, the stress has to be fairly severe; just feeling a bit anxious is most unlikely to do it.

You can often fix a milk release problem by getting your baby to feed right. For example, if your baby has not been well positioned, your nipples may be sore and you may be tense and anxious, especially if your baby is crying. Then oxytocin might not be released. Getting your baby into a correct position (remember, this includes getting yourself into a comfortable position too) so that you can feed well even once will almost always break the cycle of tension and anxiety that interferes with let-down. Work on positioning for both you and your baby, and ask for help if it is available. As soon as she is feeding well, your nipples will not be sore, you will feel better, and her strong, rhythmic feeding will cause your letdown. Then you will relax.

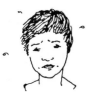

Sometimes people suggest that the main problem is that you are tense. Of course you will be anxious if you cannot get your baby to feed. The solution to a letdown problem might not be simply to try to relax; it is possible that the more you "try to relax" the more tense you will become. Some women find that gentle nipple stimulation or placing a warm wet cloth on the breast helps cause a letdown. Others say that visualizing helps; try imagining a waterfall or standing in a lovely shower of water. See what works best for your body.

It is often the case that having one good feed solves what had been a serious problem. This happens because:

- Your baby is no longer hungry and crying.

- She has learned to do it right once, so it is easier the next time.

- You have learned to do it right once, and will be more skilled the next time.

- You feel more confident.

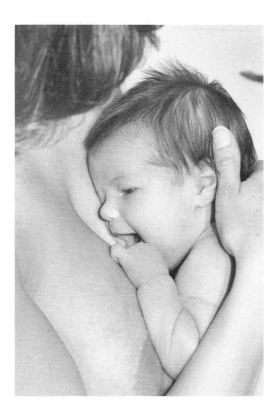

In the beginning, oxytocin (the hormone which causes milk to come down) is released in your body when your baby feeds. As your baby gets older, oxytocin can also be released when you are feeling warm and close, when you hear her cry, or when you think she might be ready for a feed (even if you are not anywhere near her!).

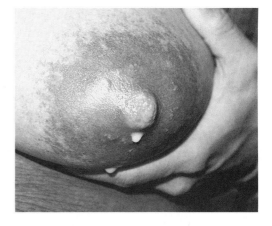

Your milk may sometimes drip from your breast when your baby is not feeding. This is the result of the letdown reflex. But don't worry if this does not happen—some women breastfeed very well without ever seeing this.

Milk and Milk Composition

☆ *Breast milk is a constantly changing food that adjusts to the age and needs of your baby.*

The composition of your breast milk is never constant. The amount of protein, fat, sugar (lactose), and other components changes. The milk you produce if your baby is delivered prematurely is different from milk you would produce after nine months of pregnancy. And that milk is different from the milk you will produce after a few months. Mothers make milk that is suited to the needs of their own babies.

The first milk your body produces is called *colostrum*. This looks yellowish and creamy. Only a small amount of it is produced, but it is exactly what is needed, and you should not need to supplement with anything else. Colostrum is high in protein and helps your baby resist infection. It also acts as a laxative, helping babies pass the thick, green/black meconium (the first stool). This is important in avoiding the development of jaundice (see pages 145–147).

In the first two or three days, your milk will gradually change from colostrum to mature breast milk. This milk is thinner and sometimes slightly bluish in color, rather than the yellow color of colostrum. Some women become anxious that their milk is not thick enough now to satisfy their babies. But in fact, it is all your baby needs for the next six months; normally, no artificial formula, water, or juice are needed.

Your body does all of this work for you, and you do not have to think about it or decide what your baby needs. But it is important to understand that the way in which you feed your baby can affect the composition of the milk that your baby takes.

Getting the Balance Right

Milk composition also changes throughout every breastfeed. The milk your baby takes at the end of a feed is different from the milk at the beginning of a feed. As you start she will get a lot of milk quickly. This milk (called the foremilk) is *high in volume, low in fat*. So although your baby gets a lot quickly, this milk is low in calories, but high in protein and other good things to help her grow and resist infection.

As your baby feeds, the composition of your milk gradually changes. After the first few minutes the *amount* of milk she gets slows down. You will see that her sucking also slows down, with longer pauses between periods of sucking.

As she sucks less frequently, she starts to get milk that is *low in quantity and higher in calories*; it is called the hindmilk. This is a gradual change that happens throughout the feed. It is not related to the timing of the letdown.

 It is essential that your baby get a good balance of both the foremilk and the hindmilk. Only in this way will she be able to take in enough milk and enough calories.

The only person who knows when your baby has had the right balance of foremilk and hindmilk is your baby.

Your baby understands her own appetite, and she knows when she is full. To ensure that she gets a good balance, therefore, all you need to do is:

- Let her feed when she is hungry.

- Let her stay on each breast until she has had enough and comes off herself.

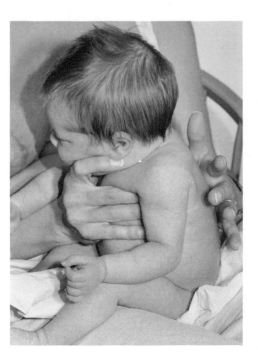

A breastfed baby is very easy to burp.

After your baby has finished one side, or if it seems like he needs to bring up a bubble in the middle of feeding on one side, sit him up so he can burp/wind. Support his chest and chin and gently rub his back. This should be all it takes to help him. Then offer him the breast once more.

The key to getting the balance right is to *let your baby finish the first breast first.* Then offer her the second side.

When she comes off the first side, sit her up. Let her burp if she needs to. (This is usually easy for breastfed babies.) Then offer her the second side. She will often take the second breast, but sometimes she will have had enough with one.

Problems that might occur in getting the balance right:

- Not positioning your baby well at your breast will result in her often not feeding long enough to get to the hindmilk.

- Limiting feeding time could cause problems for babies. Stopping her from feeding as often as she needs, or taking her off the breast after a set period of time might result in her not getting enough milk or enough calories.

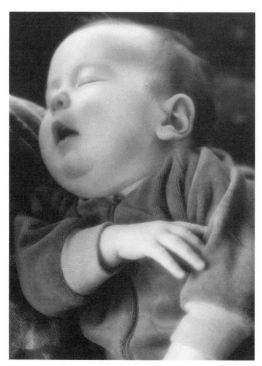

Sometimes is it very easy to tell when your baby has had enough.

Don't Impose Rules

 There are no rules about the amount of time babies need to stay at the breast.

Some babies take all they need in four or five minutes; others need forty to fifty minutes. This changes over time with each baby too; they may take longer when very young than when they are older. And there are times when they increase their feeding time over a day or two in order to boost milk production. Like adults, who sometimes eat a small meal and sometimes a three course dinner, your baby will sometimes feed for a short time, sometimes longer. Don't look at the clock to decide if she has had enough; look at your baby. Women breastfed long before clocks were invented.

Don't worry about trying to balance the foremilk and the hindmilk yourself. Your baby will tell you all you need to know. The important thing is that you do not interfere with the balance by limiting the frequency or length of feeds.

A tip: Sometimes you will need to interrupt a feed before your baby is finished. For example, you may need to answer the phone or get to the shops before they close. This is not a problem so long as you do not do it regularly. Every now and then is fine. *It is essential to keep your life normal.*

Here is a summary of what is important about milk and milk composition:

- Let your baby take a good balance of quantity and quality (foremilk and hindmilk). To do this, *do not limit the number of times you feed or the length of each feed.*

- Let your baby *finish the first breast first.* Then offer her the second side to see if she wants to take more.

Things to avoid are as follows:

- *Do not* give a fixed, small number of feeds in a day.

- *Do not* take your baby off either the first or second breast before she is finished.

- *Do not* let your baby feed if she is not well positioned.

Making Sure You've Got It Right: A Checklist

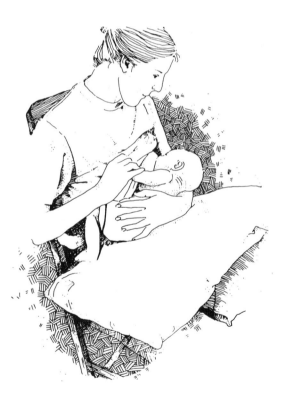

This list is a quick check over all the things you need to think about. You can find details in the previous sections if you need them.

1. *Your own posture (see pages 37–45).*

You can feed in many different positions, and you should choose the ones that suit you.

First, make yourself comfortable.

This woman is seated in a straightbacked chair, with a cushion behind her shoulders and upper back to keep her upright. It may be easiest for you in the beginning to sit in a simple, straightbacked chair.

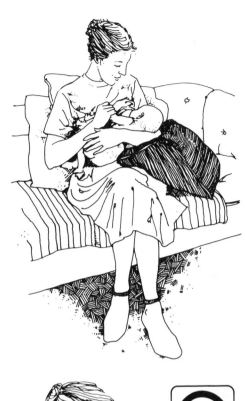

Here she sits in a deep couch. She has had to place several firm pillows behind her lower and upper back to bring her to a supported upright position. Although one leg is crossed over the other, she does have one foot flat on the floor. If her legs did not reach the floor, then she would need to put a book or cushion or box of the right height under her feet. On the other hand, if the sofa was too low and her thighs tilted upward, she would need to sit on an extra cushion. Her lap should be flat,

What do you see wrong in this picture about the woman's posture?

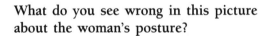

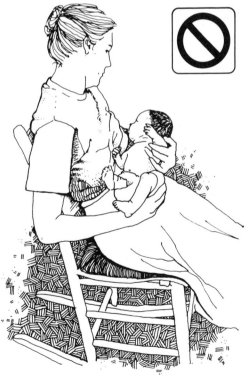

- She is slouched and leaning to one side. If she does this for long her back muscles will get quite tense.
- She is also leaning back. If she feeds like this, her baby will have difficulty taking enough breast in his mouth and her breast will tend to pull out of his mouth as he feeds.

What does this woman need to do differently?

- She needs to sit up straight in the chair, with her feet flat on the floor or on support of some other kind.
- She needs to sit back in the chair so that the small of her back and her mid and upper back are fully supported.

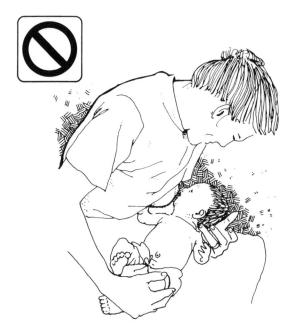

What do you see wrong in this picture about the woman's posture?

- She is hunched over her baby and her shoulders look tense. If she does this for long, she will have an aching back.

What does this woman need to do differently?

- She needs to sit up straight and let her shoulders relax. It will help if she has firm support behind her back.

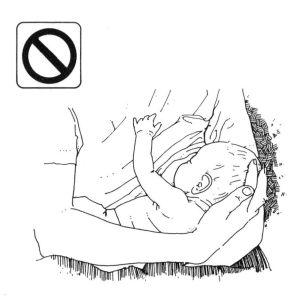

2. *Your baby's body position (see pages 46–49).*

Whatever body position you choose, you should hold your baby:

- *Close to you*
- *In a way that is well supported*
- *With his body and head facing you*
- *With his mouth just below your nipple as you prepare to feed*
- *With his head, neck, and back in a straight line*

Remember, the time you take to prepare—getting yourself and your baby in good positions—can prevent problems and even solve them if they occur.

Here, with both mother and baby lying on their sides, it is very easy for the mother to tuck the baby in close to her body and have the baby's head at the level of her breast.

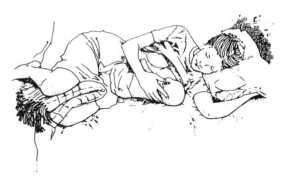

You will find this easiest to do if you start with your baby slightly lower than your breast before he goes on—with his nose level with your nipple when his mouth is closed.

The woman here is going to feed from her lower breast. If she feeds from the upper breast, then she will raise the baby up to the level of her breast with a cushion. Both her arms are then free to guide the baby to her breast.

Here is what it will look like from the side if you are feeding him while sitting up. Notice how his bottom hand is underneath his mother's breast and arm, out of the way.

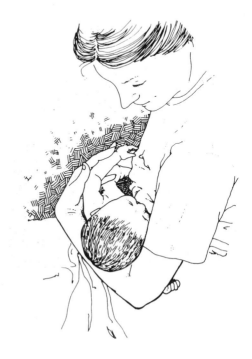

Here the baby's head rests on her forearm because she is holding him with the arm on the same side as the breast. If you use this arm, be sure he is on your forearm, NOT in the crook of your arm. We emphasize this point because bottle feeding has resulted in many women resting their baby's head in the crook of their arm. This results in the baby having to pull the breast to the side to feed.

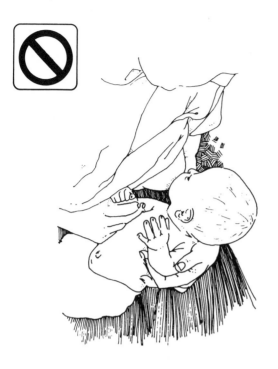

What do you see wrong in this picture about the baby's position?

- The baby is lying on his back. In order to feed he will have to turn his head sharply to one side. This will strain his neck. Imagine yourself in his position.
- The baby is not tucked in close to his mother's body. It would be difficult for her to bring him close, as his arm is in the way.

What does this woman need to do to correct her baby's position?

- She needs to turn her baby on his side facing her, place his lower arm underneath her breast, out of the way, and tuck him in close. Then he will be in a good position to begin to feed.

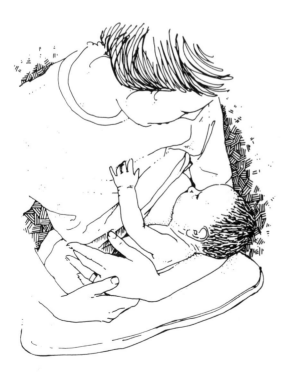

This woman has put a bed pillow on her lap to support her baby and also raise him to the level of her breast. Also notice that the baby's body and head are in a straight line. This is also important.

3. *How your baby takes your breast* (see pages 52–57).

Make sure your baby *takes* your breast; *do not* try to give it to him or push your breast into his mouth.

As your baby goes on your breast, check that he

- *Gapes his mouth wide open*
- *Takes a large mouthful of your breast*

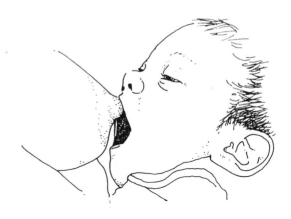

1. Position him so that his nose is at the level of your nipple, then when he gapes his mouth it will look like this picture. You will see that when he goes on the breast it is his lower jaw which does the work of taking in a big enough mouthful. His chin should end up pressed against your breast.

2. Wait until your baby's mouth is open wide —almost as if he is going to yawn—before bringing him onto your breast.

    If you wait for this to happen, then he will be sure to take a good mouthful—areola and breast tissue as well as nipple. When he takes a good mouthful, your nipple is protected from friction and will not get sore.

Sometimes your baby may open his mouth wide enough by himself. Or you may want to let your nipple brush against his lips or cheek, to show him you are ready. You may need to coax him gently with your voice. See what works for both of you.

3. As soon as you see his mouth opening wide bring it onto your breast with a quick movement of your hand (or your forearm, if his head is on your forearm).

Here is what your baby should look like when he is feeding well. Notice:

1. His chin is against the breast.

2. His mouth is open wide and the lower lip is pressed down and back against his chin.

3. His nose lies right against your breast. Notice that his nose lies on the surface of your breast and he is free to breathe. You do not need to hold your breast away from his nose.

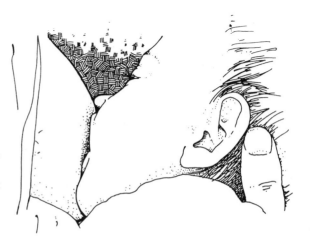

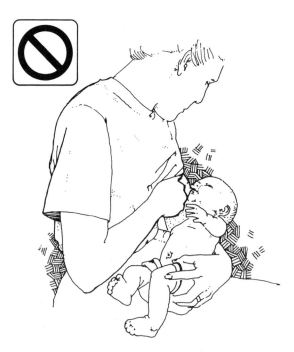

Always bring your baby onto your breast, not your breast to your baby.

In this drawing you can see clearly how the woman is actually trying to feed her baby her breast, as if her breast were a bottle. This will not work!

What does this woman need to do differently?

- First, she needs to take him off the breast immediately, so that she can try again. She needs to break the suction by placing her finger in his mouth, and then draw him off the breast completely.

- Then she needs to think about what it is that she has done and what she needs to do differently. She should go back over the points about good positioning and also read the reminders of what not to do. In this case, she should:

  1. place a pillow or something of the right thickness underneath the baby to raise his body up a bit

  2. turn his body to face hers

  3. tuck him in close

  4. wait until his mouth gapes widely

  5. bring him up onto the breast again

- If necessary (if she or the baby is very upset) she would need to calm herself and calm her baby before trying again. Some babies will go on the breast when they are crying; many will not.

It is very common today for women to bring the breast to the baby, rather than the baby to the breast. Often, even when a woman turns her baby to face her, tucks him in close, makes sure his head is level with her breast and his nose at the level of her nipple, she will then—at the last second—move her body to the baby or move her breast to the baby. If you do this (and it is so commonly done today that we feel it needs to be given special attention) then you will be off to a bad start.

If you don't bring your baby onto your breast he will not be able to take a good enough mouthful to protect your nipple and to reach your milk supply. And, once your baby is on the breast and you relax, he will actually be pulling away from your body, stretching your breast, and this will tend to pull the nipple out of his mouth or bring it to the front of his mouth. The result: sore nipples, sore breast, and a baby that is not getting enough milk.

 Helping your baby to feed well and be content is the best way of looking after yourself too.

4. *How your baby feeds* (see pages 58–65).

As your baby feeds check that he:

- *Sucks strongly and rhythmically, perhaps with occasional rests*
- *Does not hurt you*
- *Comes off the breast when he is ready*
- *During or after each feed give your baby the chance to burp/wind*

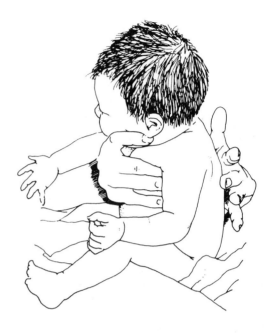

You can place the baby on his stomach, over your thigh or on your shoulder. Or you can sit him up, like this, being sure to let his chest rest on your hand and using your top finger to support his chin.

Whatever position you use, you do not need to thump your baby on the back. This can actually cause him to spit up all the milk he has taken. You may not need to do anything but sit him upright. Or you may gently rub or pat him on the back.

5. *Your baby's health.*

Your breastfeeding will be going well if your baby:

- *Grows steadily*
- *Has straw-colored (pale yellow or clear), odorless urine*
- *Has a regular, soft (but not totally liquid) yellow stool (see note that follows)*
- *Breastfeeds well, as indicated in numbers 2 and 3*

A note on your breastfed baby's stool: After the first few days of passing the greenish black meconium stool and then the brown "changing" stool, a baby who is fully breastfed should have a mustard yellow, soft (but not totally liquid) stool. It will look slightly curdled.

Babies usually settle into a regular pattern of passing stool. You will soon know your own baby's pattern, and you will see that it gradually changes over time. If there is a sudden change in this pattern (and you have not just changed your baby's diet by introducing other foods), and this change lasts longer than a day or two, watch for any other possible problems. These may be pain in his stomach or a change in color or consistency of the stool.

If all of the signs just listed are present, it is likely that your baby's health and your milk supply are fine.

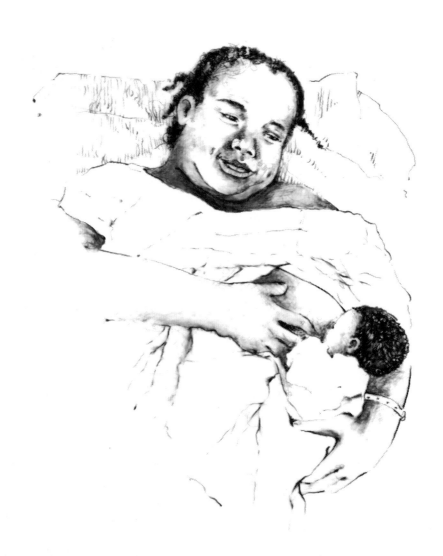

Things You Might Need to Know

Some Practical Hints on Milk Expression

You may need to express your milk for a number of reasons:

- You may have a small or sick baby who cannot breastfeed.

- You may need to be in the hospital and cannot take her with you.

- You may need to be away from your baby for longer than an hour or two.

- You may be going back to work where facilities are not available or you do not have the flexibility to breastfeed.

If you have to express a lot of milk regularly, you might want to try a hand pump or an electric pump.

There are advantages and disadvantages both to expressing milk by hand and to expressing it by pump. Briefly, these include:

1. Hand expression can be done anywhere, anytime, at no cost, with no equipment needed. Some women find they get so skilled with hand expression that they do not want to use a pump.

2. Using a good hand or electric pump properly is usually faster than hand expression. A pump that is hard to use, hurts while being used, or makes you feel sore afterward is ineffective and should not be used.

3. Hand pumps cost anywhere from $3 to $40 or more.

4. Electric pumps are very expensive. Some hospitals rent them out or lend them free of charge to mothers with babies in special care or intensive care units. In some countries pump manufacturers have arranged for breastfeeding support groups and lactation consultants to rent out electric pumps.

5. Some electric pumps can cause damage. If you use one do not choose a pump that acts by continuous suction. Make sure it cycles, that is, exerts suction and then releases it.

6. Both hand and electric pumps need to be carefully cleaned after every use. Hand expression requires only basic bodily cleanliness and thorough cleaning of milk containers.

You should decide on your method by seeing which you prefer. We will not discuss hand or electric pumps further here, as other books cover breast pumping adequately (see the resource section). You can sometimes get information about pumps from your local hospital, health professionals, or breastfeeding support group. See the resource section in the appendix for help.

We will discuss hand expression in detail, because it is free and can be done almost anywhere.

Learning to Hand Express

Many women find hand expression messy and frustrating at first. Like everything else to do with breastfeeding, practice makes it easy.

It is helpful to know that you can do this easily, without equipment, in case of emergency. *Practice it a few times before you need it.* Trying to express in a hurry before you leave your baby for the first time is not the best way to learn. Visualize this as a time to feed your baby, even if she cannot be with you. Set time aside as if you were settling down to feed.

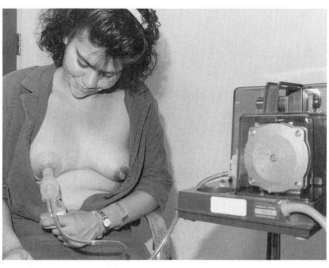

An electric breast pump, like this one, looks imposing but is actually easy to use. Many hospitals have breast pumps that any mother can use. Some have small portable ones that you can borrow and use at home.

This young mother, who has a one-week-old baby who is in the intensive/special care nursery, is able to use the hospital's electric breast pump whenever she wishes. This way her baby can receive her breast milk while he is being tube fed.

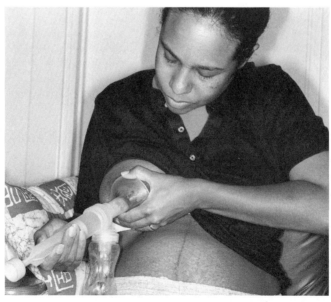

This mother, whose breasts were too full and firm for her small, four-day-old baby to grasp, discovered that using a mechanical breast pump helped. She bought the pump at a pharmacy. By taking a little milk from each breast before a feed, she made her breast softer and easier for her baby to grasp. She only needed to do this for a few feeds, while she and her baby were getting breastfeeding established.

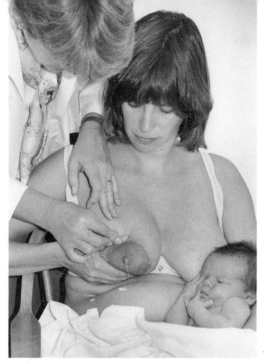

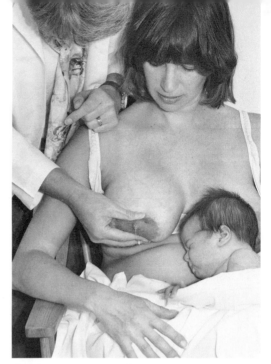

When you are learning to express, have your baby with you if possible, as this will help your milk release.

If it is not possible for your baby to be with you, then try cuddling something else— an older child, a special object—or look at a picture of your baby.

It helps to have a skilled person to teach you. If you do not have someone, then practice using the descriptions here. Remember the milk supply is well back behind your nipple.

Place your thumb flat against the upper edge of your areola and cup the rest of your hand under your breast.

Gently squeeze your thumb and forefinger together, while at the same time pressing your whole hand back and in toward your breast, to reach the milk.

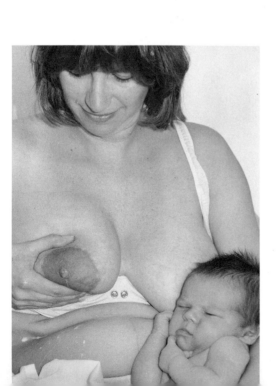

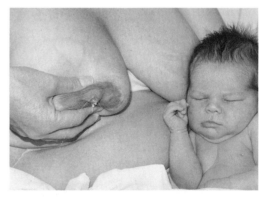

Expressing in a warm bath or shower the first few times you try might help. The warm water is relaxing, and you don't have to think about what to do with the milk. Concentrate on the expression at first, rather than catching the milk. Use some tissues or a clean cloth to catch the milk if you are not in the bath or shower. Express before a feed, rather than after; there is more milk and expression is easier.

You may find, like many women, that if you gently massage your breast first, lightly stroking down with your hand toward the nipple for a few minutes, the milk will flow more easily.

The pictures here show you the details of expression. Note that this mother is learning while her baby is on her lap. This often makes expression easier, as your letdown reflex is more likely to work well (see page 73). If you cannot hold your baby or if she is not there to look at, then try holding something else that reminds you of her or relaxes you: a blanket, a stuffed animal, your older child, whatever helps.

Many women find it helps to look at a photograph of the baby. If your baby is in a special care or intensive care unit, the staff will be happy for you to arrange to have a picture taken of your baby. Some will do it for you. (You might also tape a photograph of yourself and your family to your baby's bed in the hospital to remind the staff that your baby is part of a family.)

You can use either hand on either breast. Most women use the same hand for both breasts; their choice of hand may depend on whether they are right-handed or left-handed.

There are many different ways of getting milk out of the breast. Each mother adapts the basics to suit her body. We give just one description of how to get your milk flowing; you'll discover other ways for yourself as you become more confident.

1. Place your thumb flat on the upper edge of your areola, and cup the rest of your hand under your breast. The base of your forefinger should rest on the lower, or under, edge of your areola.

   To do this well you need to have a good handful of breast between your thumb and the rest of your hand. Feel the weight of your breast in your cupped hand. If you have a small areola, then move your fingers farther apart than the edge of your areola. If your areola is large, then move your fingers in a bit toward your nipple.

2. Imagine that milk is coming from deep within the breast through tiny tubes. Rather than pinching the tubes closed, you want to push the milk along and out. To do this, gently squeeze your thumb and forefinger together. At the same time, gently press your whole hand back and in, toward your chest.

You need to do both of these steps *together*, so that you milk the deep breast tissue as well as squeezing milk out of the ducts that lie right under the nipple and areola.

The resulting movement should feel like you are *pressing back in toward yourself*, and then letting out again, rather than squeezing.

Just as your baby makes his milking action with his lower jaw, most of the work is not in your thumb, but in the part of the hand that is cupped underneath your breast.

Some people like to think of keeping the thumb stationary while doing all the work with the lower fingers. Think of bringing the lower fingers up toward the thumb and folding your breast up, thus releasing the stream of milk.

Whichever way you do it, be careful not to slide your thumb or forefinger over your skin toward your nipple. This can cause a burning sensation. Don't be rough with your breasts: they bruise easily. Expressing should not hurt.

Once you have the movement right, your milk will take a minute or two to flow. Keep repeating the movement until you feel confident.

When you start to collect milk, simply hold a wide-mouthed container under the flow of milk. Some women have an active letdown reflex and find that the milk flow is rapid and shoots a few inches away from the nipple.

Storage of Breast Milk

Today in the United States, women are rarely advised to sterilize equipment. It may be that if you live where you have clean water and clean surroundings, then you do not need to sterilize. But it is our belief that it is best to sterilize all milk containers, storage jars, and feeding utensils, by boiling them for ten minutes. A sterilizing solution can also be used; the manufacturer's instructions should be followed. If you do not sterilize, then wash everything very carefully with hot, soapy water and rinse off the soap thoroughly. A final scalding with just-boiled water may also help.

Once you have expressed your milk, look after it carefully. If it stays at room temperature, you should use it almost immediately. It will keep in a refrigerator for twenty-four hours. In a separate freezer it can keep for a month. If you have a small freezing space within your refrigerator, do not keep it there longer than two weeks. Do not store breast milk in the rack in the refrigerator or freezer door; keep it at the back, where it is coldest.

Never refreeze milk after it has thawed, and remember not to use a microwave oven to thaw or warm frozen milk. A microwave does not heat evenly. It can overheat the milk in the center of the container and scald the baby! It also destroys vitamin C, and some studies suggest it even alters proteins.

Inverted Nipples and Nipples that Do Not Stand Out (Flat)

It is not uncommon for a woman to have one or two nipples that dip inward, like a crater, rather than stand out. These are called inverted nipples. It is also normal for a woman to have one or two nipples that do not stand out when she is cold, sexually aroused, or starting to breastfeed. These are called flat (or nonprotractile) nipples.

It is possible to breastfeed with either of these kinds of nipples, although it will be more difficult at the beginning, and you will need patience, understanding of what to do, and probably some help.

 Remember that babies do not nipple feed: they breastfeed! So right from the very first feed, encourage your baby to take a large mouthful of breast, as we describe on pages 52–65. As your baby feeds from your breast, he will draw the nipple out by his sucking action.

You may find it helpful to stimulate your nipples with your fingers just before feeding, to help them stand out. Some women like to express some milk before a feed, so that the baby gets milk as soon as he starts to suck.

Some people advise that women with inverted or flat nipples prepare their breasts in pregnancy. Two treatments are described: glass or plastic breast shells or shields that fit over the nipple and part of the breast and are worn inside the bra, and exercises to stretch the base of the nipple, using the thumbs or forefingers (Hoffman's exercises). There is as yet no evidence that either of these treatments work, and if either of them are carried out too vigorously, there is a possibility of damage to the nipples. Therefore, at present, we do not advise their routine use.

If you have problems with your baby taking your breast, and you cannot solve them, don't panic. The best thing to do is to express your milk from the side (or sides) that is causing the problem, and feed your milk to your baby by spoon or cup (see page 107).

Many women find that as their babies get bigger, it becomes easier for them to feed from inverted or nonprotractile nipples. So you might find that you express for two or three weeks, and then your baby is able to breastfeed. In this instance you may have to persist for a few days to teach him to take your breast, because he will not be used to opening his mouth wide to feed.

If you have difficulty with one breast only, it is perfectly possible to breastfeed successfully from only one side, and either express milk or not

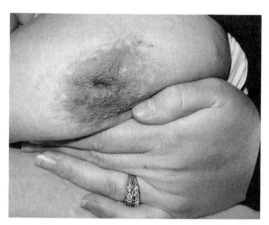

An inverted nipple dimples inward rather than protruding outward. You should still be able to breastfeed, but it will be more difficult for your baby to learn to latch on. Be patient. Be persistent. Express your milk and feed it to your baby by cup, spoon, or bottle, if you need to.

feed at all from the other side. Over time, your milk supply will adjust to your baby's needs, so that one breast will provide all the milk he needs. See the case study on pages 182–184 for an example of how easy this can be.

A Word About Your Diet

While you are breastfeeding, what you eat is important. In pregnancy your baby was growing inside you, and you were aware that you needed to eat well to help him grow and develop healthily. During breastfeeding, your baby is growing fast and depends entirely on the milk you are making.

Your body is surprisingly efficient at making milk. In fact, it seems to conserve energy, becoming far more efficient than usual during the time you are breastfeeding. So you don't really need to eat for two.

But you need to eat well to ensure that you have enough protein, vitamins, calories, and minerals for both your needs and your baby's growth. Regular meals are necessary; either two large meals each day or frequent snacks throughout the day, containing plenty of fresh fruits and vegetables. You can breastfeed successfully if you are vegetarian, but do ask your health worker for advice.

Avoid dieting during this time. You will be surprised how easily you lose the extra weight from pregnancy while you breastfeed; this is one of the advantages of breastfeeding. And it looks as if the hormones you release while breastfeeding actually help you lose weight from the buttocks and thighs, usually the most difficult places to reduce.

Contrary to popular opinion, you do not need to drink extra fluids while you are breastfeeding. Many women find, however, that they are especially thirsty, and it is always wise to respond to your body's needs. Simply drink a glass of water, juice, or other nutritious beverage whenever you are thirsty. It is a good idea to have a glass of something to drink by your side before you settle down to breastfeed.

Your baby will essentially be taking in whatever substances you take in. Think carefully about your intake of nicotine, sugar, and artificial sweeteners. Think especially carefully about your alcohol and caffeine (found in chocolate and many teas and soft drinks as well as in coffee) intake. They pass quickly into the breast milk and affect the baby in the same way they affect you.

Having these substances occasionally is fine, but regular or heavy intake will affect your baby.

Some women become so busy and preoccupied that they forget to eat or drink regularly. Neglecting your needs is not difficult to do when you are caring for the needs of a young baby, and perhaps other children as well. If this happens to you, remember that it can harm your health. You will probably continue to make enough milk, but you will become very tired. Ask others to remind you to eat, and keep food that is easy to prepare in the house.

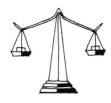

Taking Drugs or Medications While Breastfeeding

During the time you are breastfeeding, you must continue to be as careful about taking medications or drugs as you were during pregnancy. Anything you take will cross into your breast milk. Even drugs you consider harmless, such as aspirin, may have an effect on the baby. It is surprising how often we take tablets when we don't need them.

Follow this general principle: *If you do not have to take the drug or medication, don't.* This warning includes drugs like marijuana or cocaine. There are no safe levels of these drugs for babies.

Alcohol, caffeine, and tobacco are drugs too, all of which directly affect the breastfeeding baby. See the section on diet (pages 97–98). Breastfeeding women who smoke are more likely to have babies who cry a lot and develop "colic." And alcohol passes quickly into the breast milk. It has the same effect on babies as it has on us, and is harmful in regular or large doses. An occasional drink is fine, but not more.

If you have to take medication, make sure your health worker knows that you are breastfeeding, and ask her or him to explain the possible effects on the baby. Many drugs are compatible with breastfeeding. For example, if you are diabetic and take insulin every day, you can certainly continue to breastfeed. But make sure your health worker knows you are breastfeeding and helps you adjust your insulin dose accordingly.

We cannot list in this book the possible side effects of each drug. In fact, much research is still needed examining the effects of drugs or medications on breastfed babies. A new, easy-to-read book lists commonly used drugs and their possible effects when taken during pregnancy and lactation. You will find it listed in "Books You Might Find Helpful" on page 209.

If You Are Ill

If you become ill, *do your best to keep your milk supply stimulated.* During the time you are sick, *make rest and breastfeeding your priorities.* You can arrange for help around the house and go to bed if necessary, taking your baby with you. Then you can both simply rest and breastfeed.

If you need to be admitted to the hospital, try to arrange to have your baby stay with you. Sometimes you can share a room so you can be together. If your baby cannot come with you and you are well enough, express your milk regularly and send it home to be fed to your baby. If you are not well enough to do this yourself, ask your health workers or family members to help you. Remember that the painful engorgement and mastitis that could occur if you suddenly stop breastfeeding will not help your recovery.

If you do have to stop breastfeeding for a while or if your milk supply decreases, *it is always possible to restart or increase your supply.* See the section on relactation (page 108). If you have to take medications, read the section on drugs and breastfeeding (page 98).

If Your Baby Has a Handicap

If a baby is born with a handicap, parents become very distressed, especially the first few days after birth. At this time, it is hard to think clearly and to plan for the baby's feeding. Many babies with handicaps can breastfeed, and sometimes breastfeeding helps the handicap.

When a baby is born with a handicap it is common for health workers to want to observe the baby carefully. In many cases this means separating the infant from his mother. If a health worker suggests that your baby needs to be in the special care or intensive care unit, question whether his separation from you is necessary (or if you have private health care, ask for a second opinion). Make your desires to be with your baby known. If you must be separated, start to express your milk soon after birth (see pages 89–94). You may find the section on special care or intensive care helpful (see pages 102–104).

If your baby has a handicap, it will be valuable to contact other parents who have dealt with the same challenge. Many parent support groups exist, both at the local and national level. Addresses for some groups are listed in "Where to Find Help" (see page 201). Your local health workers or breastfeeding support group will be able to put you in touch with the group nearest you.

These are the principles which apply to breastfeeding any baby with a handicap:

- *Be determined that your baby have breast milk*, whether it is from your breast or by tube, bottle, spoon, or cup. The health-giving properties of breast milk, including the increased resistance to infection that it provides, are especially important for babies with handicaps.

- *Work with your baby to help him take your breast.* Find support and skilled assistance to help you.

- Even if you cannot feed from your breast, *have lots of skin-to-skin contact with your baby.*

Three of the most common handicaps with which babies are born are Down's syndrome (sometimes called mongolism), cleft lip and/or palate, and heart defects. We will discuss these here.

Babies born with Down's syndrome have decreased muscle tone, so they find it harder to support their own heads. Their bodies also have to be supported more than those of other babies. But once they have learned to feed from the breast, they can breastfeed well; and both mother and baby will benefit from the health advantages of breastfeeding and from the close contact. It helps greatly to be in touch with other parents who have faced the same situation. Contact your breastfeeding support group or a support group for parents with Down's syndrome babies; addresses are provided in "Where to Find Help." An informative pamphlet that you can obtain is listed in "Books You Might Find Helpful" (see page 209).

Babies who have cleft lip or palate can often breastfeed, though it may be difficult at first. Even if feeding from your breast is not possible, you can feed your baby expressed breast milk, making it possible for him to grow and thrive on your milk.

It is always worth trying to feed your baby at your breast. Some babies with handicaps, especially those with only a cleft lip, are able to breastfeed after they have learned to take the breast. It may help to close over the cleft with your finger to prevent the milk from escaping.

Babies with a cleft palate will find it hard to suck and swallow efficiently. You should feed with your baby in a semi-upright position and stop frequently to give him time to cope with the milk flow. Some babies benefit from using a specially designed plate that fits over the cleft, somewhat like an orthodontic plate. If your baby continues to have problems coping with the milk flow, ask for advice from your health worker, breastfeeding support group, or cleft palate association (see "Where to Find Help"). A pamphlet you may want to read is listed in "Books You Might Find Helpful." If you find it difficult to feed from your breast, or if you cannot provide all your baby's needs this way, you can express your milk and feed your baby using a bottle and teat designed for babies with clefts. Again, ask your health worker or support group for more information.

Even if you cannot feed from your breast, you can still cuddle your baby against your breast. In this way, your baby will have the advantages of drinking your breast milk from a bottle and of being close to you. Some babies with clefts will have surgery when they are slightly older to correct the handicap. Breast milk is the best way to ensure that your baby is healthy for the surgery, and cuddling is the way to keep him happy.

Babies with heart defects can also be breastfed. Recent information suggests that breastfeeding does not stress babies as much as bottle feeding. It is harder work to suck and swallow from a bottle than from the breast. So breastfeeding may be especially advantageous for babies with heart problems who need to conserve their energy as much as possible.

Jenny's story, in "Women's Breastfeeding Stories" (page 178), shows how one mother, with support from her family and health workers, successfully managed to breastfeed a baby with a particularly severe heart problem.

Remember, breastfeeding a baby with a handicap is especially valuable. He needs the health-giving properties of breast milk, and the close contact and cuddles will comfort you both.

If Your Baby Is in the Special Care
or Intensive Care Nursery

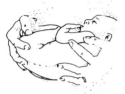

If your baby is in the special care or intensive care nursery for any reason, you will want to have as much contact as you can with him. It is especially important for both of you that you start and then maintain a good milk supply.

Breast milk from their own mothers is almost always the best food, by far, for small or sick babies. In spite of the many advantages of breastfeeding for these babies, it can be difficult to do. The routines in some special care or intensive care units are not supportive of breastfeeding. The units themselves can be noisy, crowded, and hot, and it can be hard to find a chair or get to your baby's bedside so that you can calmly touch and stroke (or just be with) your baby.

Find support from helpers who believe that your presence and breastfeeding are best for your baby. Then persist patiently, because the more your baby grows, the easier breastfeeding will become.

In summary,

- Have as much contact as possible with your baby. Cuddle him skin to skin if you can. Hold his hand or foot, or stroke him in the incubator. (If you can do nothing else, simply be with him and let him hear the sound of your voice reassuring him that all is well.)

- Start to express your milk soon after birth, and express your milk again every two to three hours after that (see pages 90–94), just as if he were with you and breastfeeding. Include a nighttime expression of milk if you possibly can.

- If you cannot be with your baby while you express milk, look at a photograph of him, or cuddle something else—a soft toy, a blanket, your older child.

- Express each time for only as long as is comfortable (or until the milk stops flowing). Remember to gently massage your breasts before you begin, and don't express for so long that you get sore.

- Ask the hospital staff if they lend electric breast pumps for use at home; it can save time if you are having to express often throughout the day.

- Tape a photograph of you and your family to your baby's crib in the hospital, so that the staff know who you all are and remember to think of your baby as part of a family.

- Ask the staff about arrangements for storage and collection of your breast milk.

- Don't worry if you get only a small amount of milk when you first begin to express it. Keep expressing frequently to build up

It is difficult to begin breastfeeding with your baby in an intensive care unit (special care baby unit). But breastfeeding, or providing breast milk for your baby, is the best thing you can do for your baby at this time. Be patient. Be persistent. Ask for whatever help you need, and keep asking if you don't get an answer that works. Take all the time you and your baby need to learn to get it right.

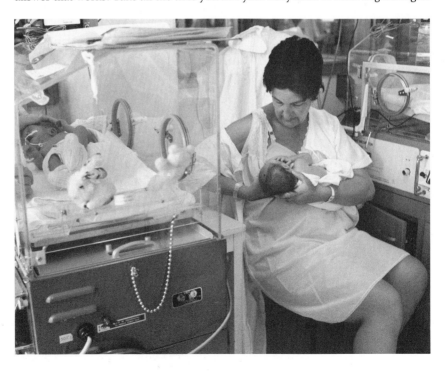

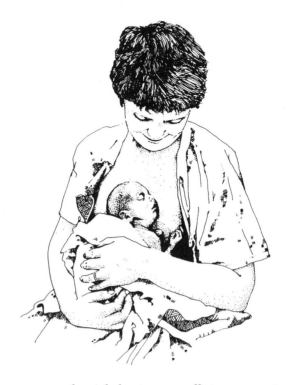

your supply. A baby is more efficient at getting milk than you are at expressing milk.

- When you first try to breastfeed, take your time, be patient with yourself and your baby, and have an understanding helper nearby. Don't be disappointed if the baby does not feed immediately. He may relax so completely in your arms that he just falls asleep.

  A very small baby can be sleepy and need a bit of stimulation to get interested in feeding. It *will* become easier for both of you as your confidence develops and as your baby gets bigger.

- Take care with positioning.

- Do not rush putting your baby on the breast.

- Let your baby feed for as long as he wants.

- If your baby stops for a while, see if he needs to burp or pass wind, and then continue.

Above all, be patient! And ask for help *whenever* you need it. You *can* breastfeed well, even with a small or sick baby.

When You Cannot Feed Your Baby from Your Breast

If you cannot feed from your breast, either for a few feeds or a few weeks, you can feed your milk to your baby in a number of ways.

If your baby is small or sick, he may need to be tube fed. The hospital staff will advise you on caring for him. The best food for him is your breast milk, even if you cannot yet feed it to him yourself.

Bottles are the most common way of giving feeds to babies, but they are not the only way. If a baby is small or has feeding problems, it may confuse him to give him a bottle teat. A baby does not have to open his mouth as widely to take in a bottle teat as he does to take in a breast, and he uses his tongue and cheeks quite differently.

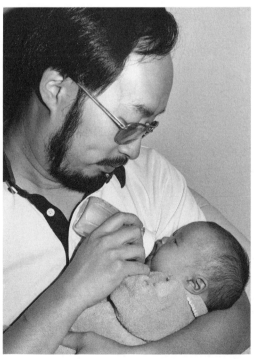

No matter how you are feeding your baby, be sure to cuddle him in close to your body. Feeding, for a baby, is as much about human contact and touch as it is about nourishment.

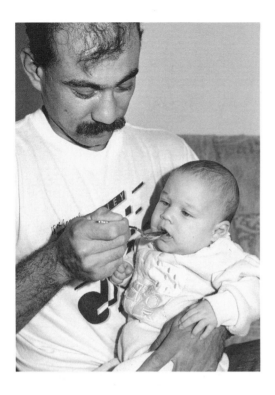

You can feed even a very young baby by spoon. When she starts to make sucking movements, tilt the spoon a little and the milk will go in. She doesn't need much for a mouthful.

This father is feeding his three-month-old daughter from a cup.

If you want to use a cup, bring it to your baby's lips, tilt it so that just a tiny amount of fluid goes into her mouth. Feed her very slowly, giving her a chance to swallow each mouthful.

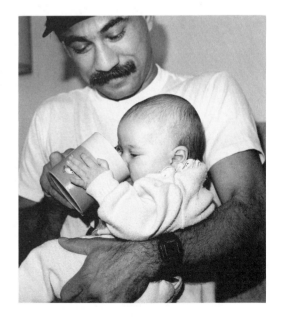

You (or your partner or helper) can feed your baby by using a cup or small glass. Simply put a small amount of milk in the cup or glass and gently tilt it to your baby's lips (see picture). Watch carefully and feed slowly. It does work!

Similarly, you can feed by spoon. Use a teaspoon and put a small amount of milk on it. Place the spoon gently against your baby's lips. When he starts to make sucking movements, tilt the spoon a little and the milk will go in. You can also try using a small dropper and gently drop milk into your baby's mouth. Be careful to do this very slowly, and watch for him to swallow before you put more in.

Whichever way you choose to feed, remember that your baby needs lots of contact with you while you do it. For both adult and baby, the experience is quite different: cuddles are as important as food.

Breastfeeding an Adopted Baby

It is possible to breastfeed an adopted baby. Though it is unlikely you will be able to stimulate your milk supply enough to fully breastfeed, *you can put your baby to your breast, enjoy her feeding, and your breasts will be stimulated to make some milk, even if you have never been pregnant or breastfed before.*

It will be beneficial to talk with your health worker or breastfeeding support group. Since breastfeeding an adopted baby is not always easy, it is useful to have support from someone who has seen it done or done it herself. If you cannot find help, the general principles are

- Make sure your baby has enough food. You can feed her by bottle, cup, spoon, or breastfeeding supplementer (see below) while you work on starting your milk supply.

- Never put her to your breast if she is very hungry, because she will become frustrated and cry. You both should associate the breast with pleasure. If she is hungry, feed her a little to calm her before putting her to your breast.

- Put your baby to your breast and let her suckle as often as you can. Pay careful attention to positioning to avoid soreness and to teach her to breastfeed properly (see pages 35–57). She probably will be used to bottle feeding, and the suckling action at the breast is different.

- Let her suckle on each breast for as long and as often as she wants. She will enjoy the cuddling and sucking, and you will have the pleasure of feeling her close to you. Stop and check your positioning if it is painful for you.

- Some women find that using a breastfeeding supplementer is helpful. This is a container for milk (either artificial milk or expressed breast milk), attached to a fine plastic tube which you can tape close to your nipple. As the baby feeds at your breast, she also feeds, through the tube, from the container. For suppliers, see the addresses on page 208, or contact your local breastfeeding support group.

- It will take some weeks for your milk supply to respond. But during this time, you and your baby have the pleasure of closeness that is not possible if you simply feed her from the bottle. Remember that breastfeeding is much more than a way to feed your baby; it is a way to give love and comfort too.

Relactating: Starting to Breastfeed After Having Stopped

You may have stopped breastfeeding and then decided you want to start again. Perhaps you were advised to stop and now find that you should have been able to breastfeed after all. Maybe you and your baby were separated for some reason and are now together; or, after weaning, your baby has become sick and you want to feed her breast milk again. You may have found that you simply miss breastfeeding.

You will be able to restart your milk supply. Most women find that even months after they stop breastfeeding they can still express some milk. It is possible to increase that supply by feeding regularly. To begin breastfeeding again, you simply put your baby to your breast as often and for as long as you can. Obviously, you will need to make sure she has enough to eat while your milk supply responds. And be careful with positioning; don't continue to feed if it hurts you. The guidelines for relactating are similar to those for breastfeeding an adopted baby, but your supply will respond much more quickly. Some women find that using a breastfeeding supplementer is helpful (see above).

What About Weaning?

It is best if you can feed your baby entirely on breast milk for the first six months. This gives your baby the best nutrition as well as protection from infection and from developing sensitivity to other foods.

Some people continue to breastfeed exclusively for longer than six months, and some babies continue to thrive on breast milk alone until they are nine months. But by this stage, many babies need to have a more varied diet. *Be guided by your own feelings and your baby's health and appetite.*

Weaning does not mean that you have to completely stop breastfeeding. You can start to give your baby extra fluids or food while continuing to

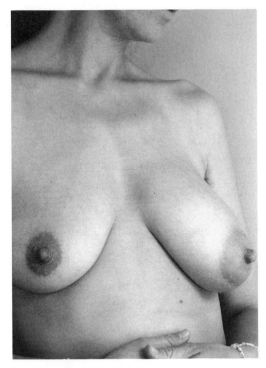

Some babies prefer feeding from one breast rather than the other. Sometimes shifting the baby's position at the breast helps, holding the baby in an under-the-arm position, so that she approaches both breasts the same way. Sometimes nothing helps, and one breast becomes larger than the other from having its milk supply always more stimulated than the other.

A woman's breasts normally differ somewhat in size and shape. Your breasts may be quite different now, but they will become more alike again when breastfeeding is over.

breastfeed. In fact some women breastfeed for over two years. They feed their babies solids and other fluids, but also breastfeed once or more a day for as long as both they and their babies want to continue.

Whether you start to give your baby other fluids or food at two or at six months, the general principle is to do it gradually. This will help your baby adjust to new foods. Equally important, it prevents you from becoming engorged. It is possible to develop mastitis if you get very full, which may happen for a few days as you cut down on breastfeeding, so watch carefully for signs of redness and pain in your breasts (see page 124).

Your baby is used to receiving all of her food from you. Some breastfed babies do not like to take bottles or food from a spoon. *Be patient and creative.* If she refuses a bottle, try a cup. If she does not like the taste of what you are offering, try something else. If you introduce food gradually and continue to breastfeed, you will feel no pressure to force her to eat more than she desires or needs.

If she does not like the new food or if she becomes sick for any reason and refuses to eat, *one of the advantages of breastfeeding is that you can return to full breastfeeding.* Simply stop giving her the extra food or

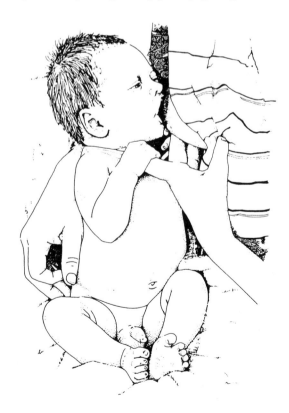

fluids and let her feed from your breast as often as she likes. Your milk supply will respond in a day or two, and you can continue to breastfeed until she has recovered from her illness. Then you can start introducing new foods again, but remember to do it gradually.

If you need to wean before six months, to go back to work or because of breastfeeding problems, *then give your baby artificial milk.* Do not be tempted to give her ordinary cow's milk, and especially not skimmed or lowfat milk. Because babies grow quickly, they must have the right balance of fat, protein, and minerals, and ordinary milk does not supply their needs. *Remember to keep all bottles, spoons, and cups clean;* even when babies are older they can still pick up infections if cleanliness is neglected.

The next best thing to breast milk is formula milk. This is usually cow's milk that has been specially modified for babies by altering the fat composition and adding the right balance of vitamins and minerals. It can be bought in most food and drugstores. Some countries subsidize formula milk for women with low incomes. Ask your health worker for further information.

As soon as you introduce food or fluids other than breast milk, your baby's bowel habits will change. Her stool, which has been sweet smelling and yellow while breastfeeding, will become firmer, darker, and more smelly. Check that she does not develop diarrhea or constipation after introducing new foods.

When introducing any new food to your baby, start with small amounts (just a teaspoon or two). Don't be tempted to continue spooning the food in, even if she seems to be enjoying it. Some babies may be allergic to a new food, and it is important to watch for signs of distress throughout the twenty-four hours after introducing the food, especially more frequent crying, more wind or gas, or skin rashes. If all is well, give her more at each feeding.

Introduce only one new food at a time, especially if your family has a history of allergic reaction to certain foods. If you give her two or three new foods at once and she becomes distressed, you will not know which food caused the problem. At first avoid foods that you or the baby's father are allergic to. It is possible that your baby will be sensitive to the same foods, so introduce these slowly and carefully.

The best guide for weaning your baby is her response to new foods. You and your baby both need to try things out and to see how each responds. Do not force her to eat foods she does not like, and gradually work toward feeding her as wide a variety of foods as you can.

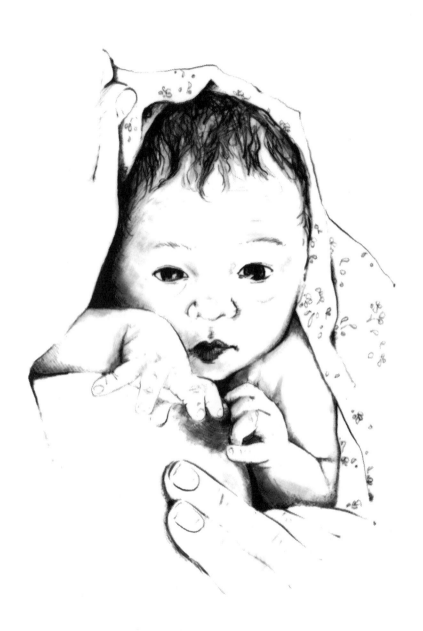

Problems: Their Causes and Solutions

Read this introduction only when you feel calm and your baby is not crying. If you need to know about a problem you have right now, turn to the list on page 121 for immediate help.

☆ ***Most problems with breastfeeding can either be prevented or easily treated.*** If a problem arises, you should try to find the cause. If you treat only the symptoms, then the problem may happen again or even get worse. Some problems may occur in the early days of breastfeeding, others after you have been breastfeeding for some time. Some breastfeeding problems occur in Western countries so often that people think they are inevitable. Babies who cry for long periods and sore nipples are two examples of this. Other problems are uncommon, and people may tell you that they cannot be solved.

☆ ***We believe all breastfeeding problems have causes.*** With understanding and skill, almost all problems can be solved. If you find breastfeeding is difficult or stressful for you or your baby, it is likely that you do have a problem. It is also likely that you can fix it. Remember that even when you are working on solving a problem, you are still continuing to breastfeed, and you are still giving your baby the best possible start in life. Some women continue to breastfeed for months even with problems, but it's obviously more pleasant for you and your baby if you can solve them.

Don't give up breastfeeding without a fight: the majority of both common and uncommon problems can be solved. But it will take knowledge, understanding, and patience.

One problem can quickly lead to another, just as in birth one intervention, such as induction of labor, can lead to another. For example, a problem with positioning may result in engorgement or a crying baby or sore nipples—or all three at once! It is important to try to prevent problems from multiplying in this way, and to treat any problem as fast as possible.

It is always better to have someone help you when you are trying to solve problems. If the steps recommended here do not help you solve your problem on your own, then seek help from the best available source. This may be the local breastfeeding support group, a health worker, or a lactation consultant. If you cannot find good help nearby, check the sources of information and help listed in the resource section.

This section will tell you how to recognize both common and unusual problems and how to solve them.

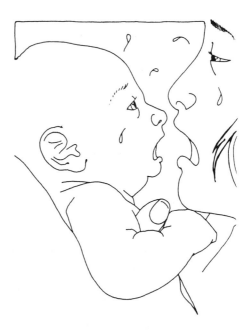

If you get frustrated and your baby gets upset, stop trying. Calm yourself. Calm your baby. Breathe. Then try again.

Home Remedies

Every culture has home remedies for illnesses of all kinds. Many are still widely used, having been passed from generation to generation by word of mouth. Many people find various home remedies helpful. The use of home remedies is a valuable part of caring for yourself and your baby, both for prevention and treatment of problems.

A home remedy is different from many of the standard products that can be bought in a pharmacy, but some over-the-counter drugs are actually botanical preparations derived from traditional home remedies. An example is senna, the plant that has been used for centuries to treat constipation and is now a major ingredient in many popular laxatives.

Home remedies can include herbal preparations, homeopathic remedies, vitamin and mineral supplements, as well as hands-on care like massage and heat therapy. Some have gained wide acceptance. For example, in many European and Latin American countries, the commonly found herbs mint (*yerba buena*) and chamomile (*manzanilla*) are regularly used for digestive ailments and whenever a sedative is needed, including treating colic in babies.

Colostrum and breast milk are used as home remedies for the treatment of several common breastfeeding problems. Some women express colostrum and spread it on sore nipples during the first days of breastfeeding (of course, we are suggesting you need not have sore nipples in the first place). Some professionals recommend the use of colostrum or breast milk as a treatment for sticky eyes in newborn babies. One home remedy that is well accepted by the general public and health professionals alike for treatment of mastitis is bed rest and an ample intake of clear fluids.

Home remedies differ markedly from culture to culture. For example, in Western thought many people swear by alternating repeated applications of heat and cold for swelling and injuries of all kinds, including breast engorgement. Warm compresses are applied for half an hour, and then ice packs. Chinese wisdom never recommends the use of cold, for either external application or in the form of food or drink, because of their belief that cold has a depressing effect on the body's energy system. In Japan fresh ginger root, grated and dropped into a large pot of boiling water, is used in hot compresses for swelling and infections of all kinds, including breast engorgement, plugged ducts, and breast infection. A treatment now prescribed in Australia by the mainstream medical community that derived from folk wisdom is the use of raw cabbage leaves held against the breast to relieve engorgement.

Scientific evidence from human or animal studies suggests that a number of home remedies may have real medical efficacy and are perfectly safe. However, there is rarely *enough* evidence to make a solid recommendation for their use. Often, little or no good research has been conducted to investigate these remedies; scientists may not know about the existence of such practices or, even when they are aware of them, may not perceive them to be of high enough priority to study.

Home remedies may take longer than prescription drugs to correct a medical problem. They often require more time and effort on your part. Some people may find them helpful, while others won't. One problem with home remedies is the question of what is the right dosage for you or your baby.

At best, a home remedy saves you money and a visit to a health worker and prevents the need for prescription drugs. For example, bed rest, fluids, and continued breastfeeding as an early treatment for mastitis is an alternative to treating mastitis with antibiotics. Antibiotics, though fast and effective, change the body's natural balance and may result in a yeast infection that will require yet another prescription drug.

Some home remedies, like vitamin C and echinacea (a common homeopathic remedy that is also the basis of a popular herbal tincture) are believed to boost the immune system and thereby aid the body's own healing response. Others that had been thought to be useful for many ailments have been proven to have negative side effects, especially if taken in large doses, such as comfrey when taken internally.

At worst, a home remedy may not work at all, may do some harm, or may delay you from getting necessary medical treatment. So, if you do try any home remedy, watch carefully for signs of improvement in yourself or your baby. Be prepared to contact a health worker if you see no signs of improvement or if new symptoms appear. We have only recommended the use of the few remedies that we feel have been tested and found to be both safe and effective.

If you are interested in the use of home remedies, ask around and be sure to check into possible side effects and proper dosages. Be careful, just as you would with the use of prescription drugs. You must be the judge of what sort of treatment you choose for yourself and for your baby. It is important to know that problems that arise in breastfeeding can quickly become more serious if they are not treated. This may occur when the woman or her health worker doesn't recognize the condition as a problem or because the proper treatment is not clear. In addition women often find it hard to take time to look after themselves, especially when they have a young baby and possibly other children or a job to handle as well.

One final warning: babies who are sick and losing weight or showing other signs such as severe vomiting or diarrhea should receive attention from a health worker.

A Word About Blame

 Problems with breastfeeding can be frustrating and painful. They are also deeply emotional.

Breastfeeding problems like sore nipples or a constantly crying baby or a baby who doesn't gain weight can challenge your feelings about yourself, your feelings about your baby, and your confidence in yourself. These problems can put stress on your relationship with your partner, and they can get in the way of developing a relationship with your baby.

We have observed that a common reaction to these deep feelings is to look for something or someone to blame. This blaming may be conscious or unconscious. It is always unhelpful.

It helps to know that this might happen, and to watch for signs of blame from other people. You might even feel a need to blame yourself sometimes.

 Be careful: *Do not let people blame you, your baby, or nature for any problems.* Problems can almost always be solved, and they *always* have a cause that can be explained.

Do Not Blame Yourself

You might be told that the problem is your fault because:

- You are too anxious, inhibited, or uptight

- You did not prepare your nipples

- You don't really want to breastfeed anyway

- Your breasts or nipples are the wrong size or shape

- You don't know enough about breastfeeding

- You don't listen to good advice

- You are continuing in spite of your baby's problems because you are doing it for your own sake

None of these is likely to be the case.

Do Not Blame Your Baby

It is sometimes tempting to think that the problem is deliberately caused by your newborn baby. You may be told that your baby:

- Is *angry*, when in fact she is hungry and frustrated

- Is *lazy*, when she is too tired, jaundiced, sleepy from drugs, or hungry to feed well

- Is *demanding*, when she cries from hunger and the need for comfort

- Has an *aggressive suck*, when your nipples are damaged from positioning problems and your baby is hungry

This is all counterproductive and untrue.

Do Not Blame Nature

Some people may blame your body for not producing the right quality or quantity of milk. Their unspoken message is that there is a basic design flaw in women's bodies, in spite of all the evidence that the

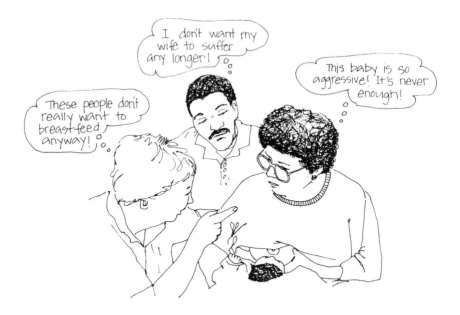

**Everyone has an opinion and
it's so easy to blame.**

human race survived very well before bottles were invented. Women today still succeed in breastfeeding wherever bottles and artificial milk are not available.

Be careful of people who tell you that:

- Your milk is too thin

- You don't have enough milk (although only a very few women really do not have enough, many women are told that this is the case)

- You have too much milk

- Your milk is too rich

- Your milk isn't good enough

This is all extremely unlikely and counterproductive.

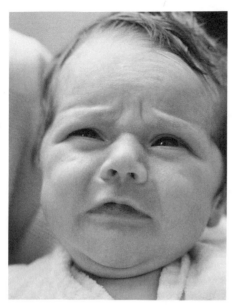

This baby looks worried. Part of parenting is learning to read your own baby's signals —different facial expressions mean different things.

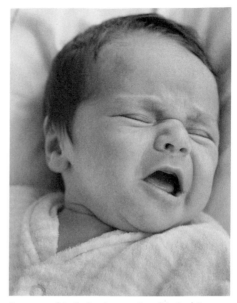

Because this baby is turning his head to the side, as if looking for the breast, it is likely to mean "I am hungry." If he has already fed well, then it could mean "I am tired and want to sleep." Over time you will be able to read his signals.

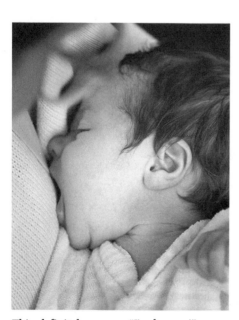

This definitely means, "I'm hungry!"

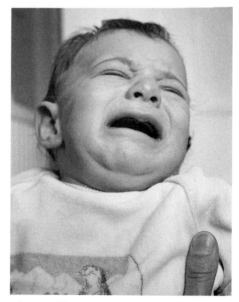

This could mean "I'm tired!", "I'm uncomfortable!", "I hurt!", or "I don't know what's wrong!"

How to Tell if There Are Problems: A List of Signs and Symptoms

Here is a list of signs and symptoms you may have if you have a problem with breastfeeding. Note that some symptoms can have more than one possible cause. It is likely that you have a breastfeeding problem if:

YOUR NIPPLES ARE

- Sore during and just after feeding (see pages 128–129, 130–131)
- Squashed and flattened just after feeding (see pages 128–129)
- Bleeding during and after feeding (see pages 128–129)
- Red and painful between feeds as well as during feeding (see pages 128–129, 130–131)

YOUR BREASTS ARE

- Swollen (see pages 123–124)
- Painful all over a lot of the time (see pages 123–124)
- Painful only in some areas (see pages 124–126, 126–127)
- Painful during or after feeding (see pages 130–131)
- Flushed (see pages 124–126, 126–127)
- Lumpy (see pages 124–126, 126–127)
- Not usually soft and feeling comfortable after feeding (see pages 124–126)

YOUR BABY

- Is restless during feeding (see pages 132–137)
- Pulls away from your breast during feeding and looks upset or cries strongly (see pages 132–137, 140–142)
- Never finishes feeding spontaneously (does not let go of your breast on her own) (see pages 132–136)
- Usually has long feeds (routinely longer than an hour) (see pages 132–136)

- Feeds very frequently (every one and a half hours or less from the beginning of one feed to the beginning of the next) *both* day and night (see pages 132–137)

- Frequently cries immediately after feeds (see pages 132–137)

- Cries inconsolably for long periods (see pages 132–137, 137–144)

- Does not pass the normal greenish black stool (meconium) in the first few days after birth (see pages 128–129, 145–147)

- Does not develop a breast milk stool (see pages 128–129, 145–147) by the end of the first week after birth

- Has a liquid stool, usually greenish in color (see pages 134–137)

- Never feeds deeply and rhythmically (see pages 128–129)

- Is not steadily gaining weight (see pages 132–136)

- Chokes or spits up because she is overwhelmed by the amount of milk she is getting (see pages 136–137)

- Remains jaundiced (yellowish skin color) one to two weeks after birth (see pages 145–147)

Problems with Milk Flow: Description, Causes, Prevention, and Solutions

It is important that your milk be removed regularly from your breast, either by feeding your baby or by expression. This is to help stimulate your supply and keep the milk moving.

Problems with milk flow may occur because:

- Your baby is not positioned well and therefore cannot milk the breast properly.

- Your milk supply exceeds your baby's demand. (This is often true for a few days after birth; milk is plentiful but your baby may not yet be feeding efficiently.)

- You may not be able to feed your baby as often as you need. Sometimes this happens if you leave the baby for a few hours longer than usual between feedings.

☆ *If you are having a problem with milk flow, ask yourself:*

1. Have I had too many visitors who want to play with the baby?

2. Are there people around who make me feel uncomfortable feeding in their presence?

3. Did I wean suddenly, for any reason?

4. Is there an obstruction to milk flow? (This may be caused by clothing, usually a bra or dress that is too tight, or by your fingers pressed into the breast when feeding.)

Problems with milk flow may lead to complications, as discussed here.

Painful, Swollen Breasts (Engorgement)

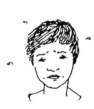

Having painfully swollen breasts (commonly known as engorgement) is usually a sign that milk is not flowing out effectively from the breast. It frequently happens between the second and fourth days after birth, and indicates that your baby and your breasts are out of balance with each other. It can also happen if:

- Your baby is not able to feed frequently

- Your baby is not feeding for long enough

- Your baby is not positioned well enough to drain the breast efficiently

As a result,

- Milk builds up in the breast

- This causes a slowdown of the blood and lymph supply

- You get painful, swollen breasts from too much milk, blood, and fluid in the tissues (edema)

To fix engorgement breastfeed well and often! Check that your positioning is right (see pages 35–45), or ask someone skilled for help.

Let your baby feed as often as she wants, and for as long as she wants. Do remember to let her feed until she is finished on the first side. She may not want the other side, but she'll take it at the next feed.

You may need to express a little milk before you start to feed: your breasts may be so full, baby cannot get a good mouthful of your breast.

For quick relief from pressure and pain, express a small amount of milk in between feeds. Try doing this in a warm bath or a shower, or after placing warm, wet cloths on the breasts.

You may be told by some helpers or friends not to express your milk. It is a common misunderstanding that expression makes engorgement worse. *This is not true.* Gentle expression helps relieve the pain of engorgement. Once you feed your baby well and express just enough to relieve the pain, the problem will resolve itself in a day or two.

If the pain is severe, and expressing a bit of milk does not relieve it adequately, you may want to take some pain medication for a very short time (usually less than one day).

Red, Inflamed Breasts (Mastitis)

If any part of your breast becomes red, inflamed, or hot to the touch, you have mastitis. Mastitis is caused principally by problems with milk flow.

Mastitis is more likely to occur when:

- You have not fed your baby as often as usual

- Your baby is not positioned well

You may have been told to use a finger to hold your breast out of your baby's way. If you have been doing this, pressure from your finger on the soft breast tissue may have blocked milk flow from that area and caused the mastitis. If your baby is well positioned, there is no need to use your finger to keep your baby's nose clear.

Mastitis commonly occurs when unusual events interrupt the normal pattern of feeding. Examples are:

- Going back to work for the first time

- Going out to an exciting event, such as a party

- Disrupting your normal feeding pattern because of travel

You may spend time organizing an event (such as your baby's christening) and look after your visitors or houseguests so you do not feed your baby as often as she needs, and mastitis may result.

Mastitis may also occur if your clothing restricts the flow of milk and blood: you may wear a bra that is tight, such as a sports bra in which to exercise, after the birth. You should choose your clothing with care.

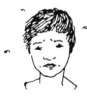

How will you know if you are developing mastitis?

1. Part of your breast may feel painful, look red, and be hot to the touch.

2. You may feel hot all over.

3. You may have chills and shivers.

4. You may feel like you are getting a flu.

Don't wait to see what happens. **Start treatment immediately so that it does not get worse.** The best possible treatment is:

1. **Feed your baby often**, and for as long as she wants. This will keep your breast milk flowing, which is the root of the problem. Gently massage any lumpy or blocked areas while your baby feeds.

2. **Be especially careful with positioning.** Find someone to help you check positioning if you can.

3. **Try expressing milk.** Some women find that expressing milk as well as breastfeeding helps to resolve the problem. But if you do this, avoid bruising your breast by too much handling.

4. **Take care of yourself (and also ask others to care for you)** as if you had a flu. Get lots of rest. Eat well. Drink a lot of fluids.

You may find it helpful to take your baby to bed with you, so that you can feed the baby often and rest at the same time.

Do not stop breastfeeding. This will make the problem worse.

Try to feed so that the part of the breast that is inflamed is drained well by your baby. This may mean that you have to feed with the baby in a different position from usual: for example, if you usually feed with the baby tucked in close to your front, then try to feed with her tucked under your arm.

If the redness and pain do not start to resolve themselves within six to eight hours after you start treatment, then *contact a health worker*. If mastitis is left to develop, a breast abscess may form (see page 127). This should never be allowed to happen. You may need an antibiotic. This will almost certainly help resolve the mastitis, but it may cause thrush in you or your baby (see pages 130–131) and should be used only when essential. Remember to complete any course of an antibiotic that you start; don't take it only until the symptoms disappear.

Blocked Ducts

Blocked ducts occur when the breast milk is not flowing well. You may feel a lump anywhere in your breast, and it may or may not be painful. This lump is milk that has thickened and is harder to drain.

This is an indication that positioning needs to be improved. Be careful to get it right at *every* feed (see page 36). You may find it helpful to try out some different positions. For example,

- If you usually feed sitting up, try lying down.

- If you normally feed with your baby under your arm, bring her around so that she is tucked into your front.

- You might also want to start with the side that has the lump for a feed or two, so that your baby feeds more vigorously on that side. Gently stroke the lump toward the nipple as you feed.

White Spots

You may see small white spots developing on the tips of your nipples. These can be due to thrush (see pages 130–131), or they can show that the openings of the milk ducts onto your nipples are blocked with an accumulation of milk solids.

Treatment is similar to that for a blocked duct:

- Be careful with positioning, and try out some new positions.

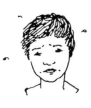

- Gentle hand expression may also help: gently squeeze behind the spot; it should pop out and free the duct. Have a warm bath or shower first, or bathe your breast in warm water.

Do not persist with expression if it is painful; instead, feed your baby well and often, and let her do the work for you. Good feeding will remove the blockage.

Breast Abscess

 Warning: A breast abscess is a problem that needs medical attention immediately.

This is a *very* rare problem and is one that should never happen. It usually occurs if mastitis has not been treated, and it is the main reason why any episode of mastitis should be treated quickly and effectively. It may also result from infection entering the breast due to nipple damage. This is a good reason to treat nipple damage quickly.

If nipple damage does not heal, then the area around the nipple may become infected. If mastitis does not resolve itself, then the red, inflamed area may become infected.

In both cases you will find that the affected area becomes very painful and swollen, and you will feel quite ill (as if you have a bad attack of flu). You will have a fever. You may also find that you are losing some pus from your nipple. Pus is a good thing, as it helps the abscess to drain (but don't be tempted to squeeze it out).

Go to your doctor, who will start you on antibiotics. The abscess will probably need to be drained surgically.

Do make sure you continue to feed your baby as often and as well as you can at this time. If you do not, then the problem may get worse. Remember that the cause in the first place was that milk was not being drained well from the breast. Even if you are losing pus from your nipple, you can still feed the baby: the pus will not harm the baby. If you do not want to do this, however, you can express your milk for a day or two, while you continue to feed from the other breast. If it is too painful to express, then breastfeeding your baby is usually the least painful way of moving milk.

It is very important that you do not wean suddenly at this time, as that would make the problem worse. If you have to go into the hospital for treatment, arrange for the baby to go in with you. If this is not possible, then make arrangements to express your milk regularly. If you have a surgical incision, you will need help to express your milk without interfering with the healing of the incision.

Problems That Cause Sore Nipples: Description, Causes, Prevention, and Solutions

Faulty Technique and Positioning

If your baby is not positioned well at your breast, a number of problems can result. These may occur in the early days as you learn about positioning. They can also occur later, perhaps because you are distracted and not as careful as usual at one or two feeds.

The most common problem that women develop with breastfeeding, especially in the first few days after birth, is sore nipples. *Sore nipples are not inevitable, and they should not occur.* It is almost always a sign that something is wrong with the way the baby is on the breast, and incorrect positioning will cause nipple damage. You may be able to see this damage as a crack on the nipple's surface or as bleeding. Sometimes the whole nipple becomes red. Perhaps you will not see any damage. But if it is sore, you can be sure that harm is being done. The soreness can usually be corrected by solving the positioning problem.

☆ *Prevention is better than cure.*

Some people will tell you that sore nipples are common, and that you should ignore them. *This is not true.* Pain is usually nature's way of indicating that something is wrong, and this is certainly the case with sore nipples.

The main cure for sore nipples is simple: get the positioning right. Read pages 36–57. Look carefully at the diagram and picture on pages 60–61. See how easy it is for your nipple to be damaged if your baby does not grasp enough breast when he takes the nipple into his mouth. The strong suction that babies can exert will quickly flatten and damage a nipple that is in the wrong place.

Remember that both you and your baby must learn about and practice positioning. It doesn't always come easily. The baby cannot help you get it right: he has a reflex that encourages him to suck strongly on *whatever* is offered to him. You need to be very careful about teaching him to take the best mouthful of breast possible.

Do not let your baby stay on the breast if feeding makes your nipples sore. Take him off and try again, even if you have to take him off and put him on three or four or more times. It is important to keep trying until you get it right.

Take the time that you need to do this. It will be easier if you can find a skilled helper. If not, then ask your partner or a friend to give you moral support while you use the pictures on page 58 to get it right.

Even if your nipples are very sore, it will not help to stop feeding and rest them. It will also not help to use nipple shields to protect them. Resting your nipples or using nipple shields simply postpones solving the problem.

Once you start to breastfeed again, your nipples will get sore again if you have not removed the cause. You may also complicate the problem by developing engorgement because you are not draining your breasts, and engorgement makes it even harder for the baby to get a good mouthful of your breast. Another complication can be that your milk supply is reduced because you don't have the regular stimulation of feeding.

Creams and lotions will not help either; some women find that they actually make the problem worse. Sensitive nipple skin may react easily to creams and lotions, and you may develop a skin problem (dermatitis) (see page 131).

If you want to put anything on your nipples, then put breast milk on them. It is high in fat and fights infection. It has no side effects and it's free. Express a few drops at the end of a feed and spread it on your nipples.

Sore nipples heal very fast once positioning is right. Sometimes after only one or two good feeds, damaged nipples are almost completely better. They should certainly be better within a day or two.

A note on babies vomiting blood: Some babies bring up a small amount of fresh red blood mixed with milk after a feed. Others vomit what looks like a large amount of blood. *By far the commonest cause in both cases is breastfeeding from a damaged nipple.* This will not harm your baby, but you will be harmed if you do not resolve the problem. Talk to your health worker. Almost always your problem will be solved by curing your sore nipples.

Thrush, or Yeast Infection

Sore nipples are not always caused by positioning. Some women develop thrush (a yeast infection) on their nipples. This can happen at any time while feeding: either when the baby is very young or when he is older. It can be caused by antibiotics. Some women are prone to vaginal thrush, and if so they may also develop thrush on the breasts.

Thrush, or yeast infection, on the breasts can cause:

- Itchy, irritable, slightly pink nipples and areolae. You may also see tiny white spots on your nipples.

- Red, exquisitely painful nipples and areolae that are sore both during and after a feed.

- Pain radiating up the breasts from the nipples, especially just after a breastfeed.

- Red sores on your baby's bottom, or white material (plaques) stuck to the inside of his mouth (oral thrush), or white spots on the back of his throat.

Thrush can happen after a period of trouble-free feeding. If you are prone to thrush, you should be especially careful while breastfeeding. It can be one side effect of using antibiotics for yourself or your baby, as it disturbs the normal balance of microorganisms in the body. Watch carefully for signs of thrush if you use antibiotics.

If you have thrush it is important to treat both yourself and your baby. It is easy to keep reinfecting each other if you do not. It is also important to treat it quickly, as it can be very painful for you (it is rarely painful for the baby). It can be treated efficiently and well.

Treatment of thrush is as follows:

- Ask your health worker for a prescription or medication to treat thrush. This should be an antifungal treatment (nystatin or miconazole are the generic names of two medications). You will need to treat both your nipples and your baby's mouth. You may also need to treat your vagina and your baby's bottom.

- Spread the antifungal cream on your nipples and your baby's bottom, and put the medication into your baby's mouth (on the white patches), using a cotton pad or dropper. Leave your baby's diaper off for a few hours, if you can, if he has a sore bottom.

The treatment should work in one to three days.

- If the infection is resistant, you or your baby may need to take oral treatment, which works on the whole body (systemic treatment). This is usually needed to treat radiating breast pain, which will take about a week to resolve itself.

Men can have thrush and show no symptoms. If the infection recurs after treatment, make sure all of you—baby, partner, and yourself—are treated the next time.

There is a very sound theoretical basis for the use of a home remedy, bicarbonate of soda (common baking soda), to treat thrush both on the mother's nipples and in the baby's mouth. If you wish to try this, place 1 tsp of baking soda in 1 cup (230 ml) of sterile water or water you have boiled for 20 minutes. If you put the solution in a jar with a tight lid, you can keep it with you and use it for as long as necessary. Each time you use it, shake it up and moisten a clean cloth or cotton swab. Use the solution both on your nipples and on the inside of your baby's mouth. You can try to rub off some of the white material on the baby's tongue and gums, but be very gentle.

Dermatitis, or Irritation of the Skin

Some women develop an inflammation of the surface of the nipples, sometimes extending to the areolae, while breastfeeding. This can occur at any time. It is usually caused by a reaction to something that you have put on your nipples, such as a cream or ointment. It can also be caused by contact with clothing or sensitivity to a soap or detergent you use to wash clothes.

Removing the cause of the irritation may be all that you need to do. Stop using the cream, keep only soft cotton fabrics or silk next to your nipples, change your detergent. Use air to dry your nipples after bathing.

In the very rare cases where the irritation does not resolve itself, ask your health worker for a prescription for hydrocortisone cream, 0.5 percent. This should be applied *very* sparingly for only two or three days, and you should gradually reduce the number of times you apply it. Do not stop the treatment abruptly, because if you do the problem will recur.

Problems of Milk and Milk Supply: Description, Causes, Prevention, and Solutions

Not Enough Milk

Today, when there is so little confidence in breastfeeding in many cultures, almost all women wonder at some time whether they have enough milk for a baby. Some wonder because their babies are not gaining weight as quickly as the charts say they should. Some women doubt their milk supply if their babies cry a lot. Others wonder if their babies want to feed more often or longer than "normal."

So it is not surprising that not having enough milk is often the reason given by women for stopping breastfeeding or for supplementing their feedings. In fact, some studies have found that as many as 75 percent of the women who stop breastfeeding do so because they feel they do not have enough milk to feed a baby!

Only a tiny percentage of women (probably about 1 percent) are truly not able to produce enough milk to feed their babies. For most mothers and babies, the causes of insufficient milk are both *preventable* and *treatable*. After all, these women's bodies sustained their babies' lives during pregnancy; why should their bodies become incapable of sustaining their babies' lives after birth?

It simply does not make sense that so many women would be incapable of making enough milk. If this were the case, the human race would not have survived all the years before artificial baby milks were invented. Instead, it is likely that when a baby does not receive enough milk it is for a reason that can be corrected. Causes of insufficient milk are most likely to be problems with positioning or problems with milk flow, both correctable problems.

If your baby is not well positioned at the breast, then she will not be able to take enough milk to satisfy her hunger. And because the amount of milk your body makes depends on the amount of milk your baby takes (see pages 71–74), you will not make enough milk, because only a small amount is being taken from your breasts.

There is wisdom in the body. It tries to make only as much milk as is needed. That is why the quantity of breast milk can go up and down according to the baby's changing needs. It is also why, when supplements are given to babies, women's bodies respond by making less milk, as their babies take less from them.

Similarly, if a baby is not able to feed often enough, or for as long as she needs, then the woman will not make as much milk as her baby needs. So it is likely that women who have not had enough help with positioning their baby correctly, who have been taught to limit their feeding times, or who give supplementary bottles will not produce enough milk. The result is a dissatisfied, crying baby who does not gain weight well, even though she may be at the breast almost constantly. This baby may not wake for a feed or may fall asleep immediately after starting to feed because she is hungry and not getting the food she needs.

Insufficient milk is almost always a problem that can be treated. It is best if you start to treat it soon after you suspect a problem, rather than waiting until both you and the baby are tired and frustrated and you are anxious and your baby is hungry.

To treat the problem of not having enough milk:

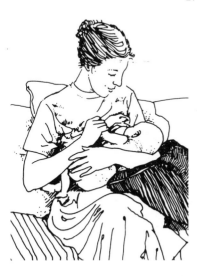

1. **Check your position and that of your baby carefully.** For some women and their babies, even a small change of position matters. So check the photographs and drawings carefully and compare them to the way your baby looks while on the breast. Don't forget to check your own body position too. Sometimes, when you are anxious, you might concentrate more on your baby, when the problem could actually be solved by moving yourself a bit more upright. This makes it easier for your baby to grasp a bit more of your breast in her mouth.

   Some babies can feed well, and some mothers can make plenty of milk, even if the positioning is not quite perfect. But there are some mothers and babies who seem to need it to be *exactly* right; these babies are often small babies, who tend to be sleepy and slow to suck. If they have exactly the right mouthful of breast tissue they do well, but if the positioning of either mother or baby is not exactly right, then they tend not to respond and not suck well.

   Getting the position exactly right is also important for some women who have large, soft breasts (see page 00 for what to do). It really is worth persevering to solve this problem. The most important things are patience, time, and an understanding of the ways to get positioning right.

2. **Encourage your baby to feed as often, and for as long, as possible.** This may be very often for the first two or three days after you start to treat the problem, because your baby will be hungry, and it will take a day or two for your breasts to respond to the increased demands. If you can arrange to have help in the house, then do so: you may find it best to go to bed with your baby, and feed as often and for as long as you can for a couple of days. Make sure you are careful with positioning at each feed.

It is important to have confidence in your body: it *will* respond, but it will take a couple of days before you really see the results and probably one or two weeks before your breasts and your baby are really in balance.

Think carefully before giving supplements to your baby at this time. It is a difficult decision to make, because your baby is hungry; but supplements do make it harder to produce milk. On the other hand, if the problem of insufficient milk is longstanding, and there is concern that your baby is not gaining enough, then careful supervision by a skilled person is needed. The treatment is still as previously described, but there may be a need for careful supplementation for the baby too. If so, you may need to express as well as breastfeed as much as possible, to stimulate your supply.

Foremilk/Hindmilk Imbalance

Some women find that their babies have problems that don't make sense. These include:

- Baby crying inconsolably either just after feeds or between feeds

- Baby pulling off the breast and acting unhappy while feeding

- Baby having a greenish, liquid stool

- Baby not gaining weight well

- Baby wanting to feed for long periods: an hour or more at each feed

- Baby wanting to feed very frequently: more often than every two hours from the beginning of one feed to the beginning of the next, day and night

- Baby growing well, but not content

These problems, which often occur in combination with each other, lead some women to believe they do not have enough milk to feed their babies. This is almost never the case.

The real problem is probably that the baby gets too much foremilk at the beginning of the feed, and not enough hindmilk (see pages 76–78). So the baby gets enough quantity, but not a balanced quality. She gets too few calories, and she is hungry and wants to feed more often. She may also get too much sugar (lactose), which can cause distress and a loose green stool.

This problem may happen when the baby does not have enough breast in her mouth or when the mother restricts breastfeeds and takes her baby off the breast after a set time. It seems to occur most commonly in mothers with an abundant milk supply.

Examples of situations that might create a foremilk/hindmilk imbalance are:

1. Imagine that you have been told to take your baby off the first breast after five or ten minutes and put her on the second side. She may not have reached the hindmilk on the first side yet. She will still be hungry and will feed well on the second side, but will get a second helping of low-calorie foremilk, rather than the high-calorie hindmilk that she needs. She will come off the second side, having taken a lot of milk, but without the right balance of foremilk and hindmilk. She may not have reached the hindmilk on the second side because she got too full.

   She will be hungry soon after feeding, in spite of the fact that she seems to have fed well. What she needs is calories! She will want to feed frequently and may not gain weight well, in spite of the fact that she is taking lots of milk.

2. Imagine that you have been told to feed from only one breast at each feed. You let her finish the first side and then stop. But your baby may still be hungry, and need some foremilk from the second side. She may even need both the foremilk and the

hindmilk from the second breast. She too will still be hungry and will want to feed often. She may not gain weight well, yet appear to be feeding fine.

The best judge of the timing of each feed is your baby. Only your baby knows when she has had a good balance of foremilk and hindmilk, and when left to her own devices, she will always come off the breast herself in due time, provided she is feeding correctly.

Treatment of this problem is simple:

- Check to be sure positioning is correct.

- Let your baby feed for as long as she wants on each breast.

See pages 76–79 for more information.

Too Much Milk (Oversupply)

A small number of women find that they produce too much milk for their babies. You may have this problem if all or most of the following occur:

- Your breasts normally get full and tender between feeds, even after several weeks of breastfeeding.

- Your baby brings up more than one or two mouthfuls of milk after almost every feed.

- Your baby gains weight very fast.

- You leak milk to the point that your clothes are almost always wet.

- Your baby gets distressed while feeding, especially each time she begins to feed.

- Your baby pulls away from your breast during the feed, choking and spitting.

- Your baby has a normal but plentiful stool.

If your problem is too much milk, you will have most or all of the symptoms just listed. It is easy to confuse oversupply with a foremilk/hindmilk imbalance (see pages 76–79). But if you have most of the symptoms just listed, then it is likely that oversupply is the cause, and you truly do have too much milk.

Note: The problem may be temporary, easing up when your supply adjusts to your baby's needs. So it is worth waiting one to two weeks to see if the problem resolves itself on its own.

Do not be tempted to take your baby off the first breast and put her on the other side just to relieve your fullness. All she will do is take high-volume foremilk from both sides, without getting to the low-volume hindmilk on either side, and the problem will continue. You will go on producing too much milk and she will be unable to satisfy her appetite with foremilk alone. Instead, express just enough to feel comfortable. This small amount of expression may also make it easier for her to start to feed without being overwhelmed by the amount of milk.

If the problem persists, then it may be worth deliberately feeding from only one breast at each feed. In this way each breast will be stimulated only at every second feed, and the milk supply will soon be cut back accordingly.

Babies Who Cry A Lot:
Causes, Prevention, and Remedies

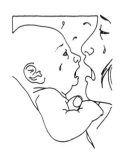

One of the hardest problems for parents to deal with is a baby who cries a lot. Crying is your baby's only way of trying to communicate what he needs and wants. Crying indicates a need, which may be:

- Hunger.

- Pain.

- Emotional distress.

- Physical discomfort.

- Overstimulation (when we are exhausted, we are likely to feel like crying!).

Sometimes it is not possible to satisfy the need and pacify the baby, but it is always important to try to work out what the cause may be in case you can help.

Over time you will learn the difference between your baby crying because of hunger and crying because of other reasons. The learning is a matter of trial and error.

One of the problems that has arisen from the common use of the term *demand feeding* (a term we never use in this book) is the mistaken idea that a baby needs to feed every time he cries. In fact, babies have a number of reasons for crying, and feeding is not always the answer.

It is almost always possible to calm an older baby by putting him to the breast, but a newborn will usually feed well only if he is hungry. If he is not hungry, he may fuss at the breast and possibly cry even harder. It may be worth trying, but do not persist if he is not interested.

The other problem with the term *demand feeding* is the mistaken idea that babies always cry when they are hungry. In fact, some babies do not cry when hungry. If you have a very quiet, sleepy baby, who is not interested in breastfeeding you will have to make sure that he feeds as often as he needs. Unusual quietness or sleepiness happens most often in the first few days after birth if:

- Your baby is small or sick

- You had medication during labor or an anesthetic (drugs affect the baby longer than they affect you)

- Your baby is jaundiced

It is unlikely that the sleepiness and disinterest in breastfeeding will persist after the first week, but it is important in these circumstances to feed your baby often, with no longer than five to six hours between each feed.

Working Out Why Your Baby Is Crying, and What to Do About It

The first question to ask yourself is, *When* does my baby cry? If it happens immediately after a good feed, then he is unlikely to be crying from hunger. He may be crying because of wind or gas or the discomfort that comes before passing a large bowel movement. Or it may be that in the early days after birth, as he adjusts to the feeling of a full stomach, he feels uncomfortable for a short while after feeds.

If any of these are the reasons for crying, then one or more of these treatments may be useful:

- Burp your baby (just hold him in an upright position and the wind or gas should come up easily).

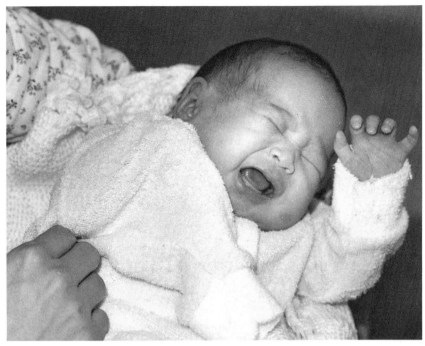

Many parents find the most difficult part of parenting to be coping with a young baby who cries and cries and cannot be consoled. Babies communicate many things through crying; it is not always easy to find the cause. People often call this kind of crying colic.

- Hold and comfort him.

- Check to see if his diaper or nappy needs changing.

- Cuddle him quietly. Try different positions: upright or on his tummy. Always tuck him in close to you. A baby sling that holds him close to you might help.

- Swaddle him in a wrap or blanket. Tuck his arms across his chest and wrap him firmly, so he is warm and secure.

Sometimes playing calming music, and walking the baby in rhythm to this helps. Your baby may respond to being cuddled and stroked in a warm bath. (Before getting in the bath with the baby, make sure it is not too hot for him: test the water on the inside of your wrist.) Or he may respond positively to gentle humming in his ear, especially a low note. (Try humming a single note for a minute or so.)

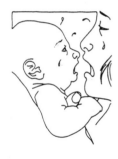

Sometimes a crying baby just will not stop, no matter what you do. Just let him cry but stay with him, cuddle him, and don't let him feel abandoned. Sometimes this will be hard to do; you may feel frightened of him or angry at him. If this happens, then ask for help with your baby from another caring adult.

A baby who cries after a feed and does not respond to your efforts may be indicating that there is a problem with the timing of the feed. This may happen if you have been advised to take the baby off the breast after a fixed period of time.

This can cause two problems:

1. He may not have had enough milk, and may need to be left on the breast longer.

2. He may not have had enough hindmilk, which he should get toward the end of the feed.

Although your baby does not need much hindmilk, it is important that he get the high-calorie hindmilk as well as large quantities of the foremilk. This is explained on pages 76–79.

The solution to these problems is simply to leave your baby on the breast for as long as he wants (see page 79). If he takes a long time at each feed (regularly taking more than fifty to sixty minutes), then check the positioning (see pages 35–49), because it is possible that he is not feeding as efficiently as he could.

Sometimes a baby who has had repeated difficult experiences at the breast will cry in obvious distress when put to the breast. This baby is responding in the only way he knows how to the fact that he has learned that breastfeeding is frustrating.

This baby needs to learn that being close to the breast is pleasurable. He also needs to experience a good, satisfying feed. Imagine if every mealtime was painful for you. You would soon learn to dread mealtimes and not want to eat, and you would lose weight rapidly. The same is true for a baby.

It is important to prevent this problem if you can. This is another reason why it is so important for the baby to have a good experience at every single feed, right from the first feed: this way he will learn that feeding is pleasant and easy.

Remember to cuddle and calm your baby before you try to feed. Otherwise he learns to associate your breast with distress.

If this problem has developed, then remember that two things are important:

1. Both you and your baby must learn to associate contact with the breast with warmth and pleasure rather than pain and frustration.

2. Your baby needs to feed well and continue to gain weight.

Ways of solving this problem include the following:

- When you and your baby are both calm, take time to be with him. When possible, lie down with him next to you, with skin-to-skin contact. Keep him well cuddled into your breast, so that he can see, feel, and smell it. Do not try to feed him if he is not interested. Just cuddle and stroke him.

- Make sure he has enough food. If it is impossible for him to feed well at the breast, then you need to express your milk to keep your supply going (see pages 89–94) and feed this milk to your baby by spoon, cup, or bottle (see pictures of how to feed using these methods, page 106).

- Once he has learned that the breast is a comforting and plea-surable place to be, and his hunger is satisfied, you can bring him back to the breast. This should take only a few hours and a couple of good feeds. It is usually best to do this when he is

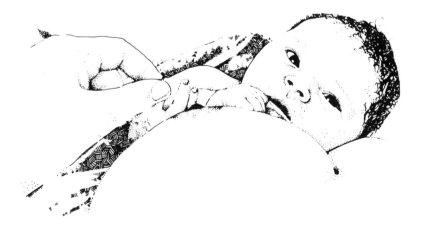

not very hungry. If you can, have some help available for positioning him. Hold him close to you, encourage him to open his mouth wide, and move him onto the breast as shown on pages 64–65. Some people find it helps to express some milk into the baby's mouth before he goes on; the taste reassures him. Don't persist if he cries; just cuddle and stroke him until he settles down, and then try again.

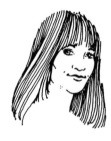

Remember to take a few slow, calming breaths and do anything else that calms you before attempting to feed. Soothing music can help put you in a relaxed mental state. Often it takes only *one* good feed for you and your baby to feel quite different about breastfeeding.

If your baby will not be comforted and cries hard for long periods with no apparent cause, don't despair. It is likely he would behave the same way if you put him on a bottle. Find support for yourself and keep looking for the source of the crying. Others may have helpful suggestions. At the worst, and if nothing else helps, then sit tight until he is three or four months old, at which time this type of crying (sometimes called colic) often disappears.

Food Sensitivity (Allergy/Intolerance)

Sometimes a baby cannot be comforted easily either after a feed or throughout the day because he has developed a sensitivity to a food that you are eating. Traces of this food pass through the breast milk to the baby. A baby can be allergic to any food. Some people will advise you not to eat certain foods when breastfeeding. But, in fact, food sensitivity differs from one mother and baby to another. It is impossible to generalize from someone else's experience.

If you are concerned that your baby may have food sensitivities, then ask yourself the following questions:

- Does my baby cry inconsolably for long periods?

- Does my baby find it difficult to settle down and sleep for any length of time and look anxious and unhappy much of the time?

- Does my baby have any other signs of sensitivity, such as rashes, dry, rough skin or eczema, or a raw-looking bottom after passing a stool?

- Has my baby been given any formula or other food or drink that might have contained something to which he is sensitive?

- Have I tried to investigate all of the other possible causes of this crying?

If you find you cannot help your baby's crying by any of the ways already described in this section, then explore three other areas:

1. Do you smoke?

2. Do you drink coffee or other caffeinated beverages?

3. What do you eat?

Recent evidence shows that women who breastfeed and smoke are more likely to have babies with inconsolable crying, or colic. This happens because substances from smoking are passed into the breast milk. It may be worth the effort to stop smoking to have a settled baby. Don't expect the crying to stop immediately; it takes a few days or more to remove the toxins from your body.

A high intake of caffeine by breastfeeding women seems to be linked with excessive crying of their babies. Monitor the amount of coffee and tea you drink, and remember that many soft drinks contain caffeine too. Try cutting down on these beverages and drink water, fruit juice, or herbal tea instead. Many soft drinks now have caffeine-free versions. Again, you are unlikely to see immediate changes in the amount your baby cries when you stop or cut down your caffeine intake. It may take a few days for the caffeine to stop affecting your baby.

Next take a careful look at your diet. It is best to do this with skilled help, as any diet is complex. To start looking at your diet, ask yourself the following questions:

- Does anyone in my family or my partner's family have allergies?

- Was I bottle fed in infancy or given solids very early?

- What foods have I eaten in the past two days? (It takes varying amounts of time for food to enter your bloodstream and then your milk.)

  If you keep a diary of foods eaten for the two days prior to when your baby has a bad bout of crying, it may be obvious what food to suspect.

- Am I eating any food that I do not really like, but that I think is good for the baby?

   An aversion to a certain food is often a good indication that your body has a problem with that food. If that is the case, it is not wise to force yourself to eat it. It is not uncommon for women who are pregnant or breastfeeding to drink extra cow's milk, up to a pint or two a day. They may do this even when they do not like milk and do not normally drink it because they believe it is good for their growing baby. This can then cause problems for the baby, who may be sensitive to cow's milk as a result of the mother's sensitivity.

   The mother herself may have symptoms that worsen; for example, headaches (including migraine headaches) or skin symptoms.

- Am I eating particular foods for which I have regular cravings?

   You may, conversely, develop a *craving* for a food to which you are allergic, such as eggs, peanuts, or chocolate. If your body is not handling a certain food well, your baby may become sensitized to it.

If you suspect a specific food sensitivity, try eliminating the most likely food for a week or two. You should notice a difference in your baby by then. Sometimes the baby's behavior may get worse for a day or two before it gets better. This is because of withdrawal; the baby will then improve after a week or so.

If you elect to cut out foods you suspect may be a problem, cut out only one kind of food at a time. If, for example, you suspect that you are sensitive to cow's milk *and* eggs, then cutting out both of these might solve the sensitivity problem, but it will not tell you which food is causing that problem. Cutting out a number of foods also makes it harder to eat a balanced diet. The more food you eliminate, the more difficult it is to balance your diet.

Other Problems:
Description, Causes, Prevention,
and Solutions

Jaundice

Jaundice occurs when the baby's body finds it hard to break down, or get rid of, a substance called bilirubin. Bilirubin is yellow and this is why babies look yellow when they are jaundiced. They have too much bilirubin in the bloodstream. The higher the level of bilirubin in the blood, the more yellow the baby looks.

The aim in treating any form of jaundice is to get the bilirubin level down to a normal level.

Jaundice is common and sometimes reaches higher levels in breastfed babies. A breastfed baby often will take longer to get rid of the greenish black stool (meconium) that is in the newborn's gut than a bottle fed baby will.

If breastfeeding is limited in frequency or duration, or if the baby is not well positioned, then he will not take as much colostrum or milk as he needs, and so delay passing his meconium.

Meconium is rich in bilirubin, and it seems to get reabsorbed into a baby's body if he does not pass it quickly. Colostrum, which your breasts produce in the first day or two after birth, has a good laxative action and will help your baby to pass stool at the right rate for a breastfed baby.

It is likely that jaundice is actually *caused* by some of the inaccurate feeding advice that has been given for so long, especially advice that has limited the amount of colostrum and breast milk that babies have had in the first few days.

To prevent and to treat jaundice, which is usually at its peak on the first, third, or fourth day after birth, your baby needs to:

1. Breastfeed soon after birth,

2. Breastfeed well, and

3. Breastfeed whenever he wants right from the first feed.

Often it is recommended that a baby be given extra water or glucose to help with jaundice. This is not useful and is likely to slow down the establishment of your own milk supply (see pages 71–75). Breastfeeding well is often all that is needed to eliminate the jaundice. Water or glucose solution may actually increase the problem of jaundice, because they do not contain the protein that your baby needs. Giving these fluids also reduces the stimulus you need for your breasts to make milk.

Other people may suggest that you wake and feed your baby every three hours. This may not help. Babies feed well only when hungry. You should concentrate on making every feeding as effective as possible, and feeding when, and for a long as, your baby wants to. If your baby is sleepy (as is common with jaundiced babies), you may need to wake him. But do not try to force him to feed from your breast. If he will not feed from your breast, express your milk and encourage him to take this breast milk by cup, spoon, or bottle.

Often, having one or two really good breastfeeds will immediately improve the jaundice.

A health worker may suggest phototherapy (light treatment) for your baby if the bilirubin level is high. You might want to get a second opinion to see whether phototherapy is really needed, as it is sometimes prescribed for even mild jaundice. In suitable climates some mothers choose to sit in the sun to breastfeed to expose the baby to the benefits of sunlight, rather than phototherapy light. *If you do this, take care to avoid sunburn.* If your baby is put under a bilirubin light, then be especially careful with feeding. Babies can get dehydrated as a result of phototherapy (they get diarrhea). This is a case where extra water might be necessary to treat the dehydration, especially if the phototherapy is continuous. If so, express milk in addition to breastfeeding, to keep up your supply. Breastfeed as often as you can.

Jaundice can also occur if:

- Your baby was born prematurely

- Your baby is bruised, perhaps as a result of a difficult delivery

- Your baby has an infection

In any of these cases your baby should be cared for by a pediatrician. In all cases the best thing you can do is give your baby your own breast milk, either directly from your breast or after expressing it.

Remember that it is important to stimulate your milk supply and keep your milk flowing. If you cannot breastfeed directly, express your milk. See pages 89–94.

 Jaundice should never result in problems with breastfeeding. Instead, breastfeeding is usually the best treatment!

The most uncommon cause of jaundice is called breast milk jaundice. In this case the baby reacts to a substance in the mother's breast milk or the mother lacks a substance in her milk. As a result the baby becomes jaundiced. This will happen after the first week, not in the early days. *This type of jaundice usually stays at a level that is noticeable but not dangerous.* The level falls gradually throughout the next several weeks. Since the jaundice will disappear of its own accord, you do not need to do anything different—just continue to breastfeed.

Until the level starts to fall, it is important to have the jaundice monitored by a health worker.

Some people may advise you to stop breastfeeding. This is almost never necessary. If the jaundice level becomes very high, then interrupting breastfeeding for a day or two while you express milk and feed your baby alternative milk (either donated breast milk or artificial milk) will be helpful.

Blood in the Milk

In the early days of breastfeeding, some women find that they have streaks of blood in their breast milk. It can come from one or both breasts. There is no pain or nipple damage associated with this.

This seems to be the result of the extra growth of the ducts during pregnancy. It will resolve itself in the next few days. Most women never notice what is happening unless the baby vomits.

Just keep breastfeeding, as the blood will not harm the baby. His stool may be a darker color than normal, and if he vomits or spits up there may be dark flecks in the milk. Do not be alarmed.

If the blood persists for more than a week, then contact a health worker. It is possible, but highly unlikely, that the bleeding indicates a more serious problem.

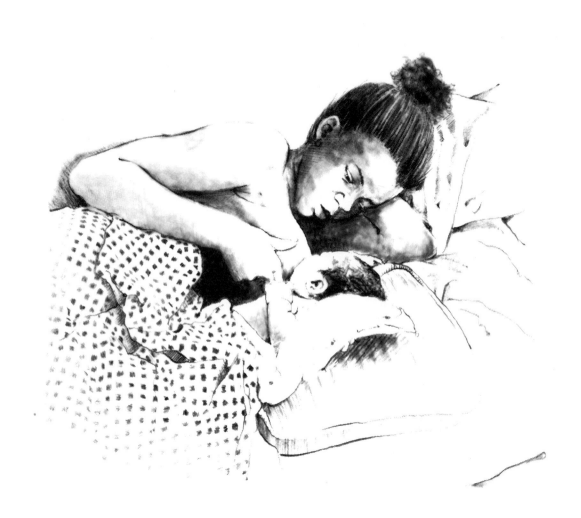

Why Women
Have Problems with
Breastfeeding

As we said before, most problems with breastfeeding can either be prevented or easily treated. Once women develop problems they often find that they are on their own. In many countries there is little support either from family (who often do not know the answers) or from health workers (who often do not know the answers either).

The fact that most breastfeeding problems are preventable or can be treated is not widely known by mothers or health workers.

Why is this?

The reasons why so many women today have problems with breastfeeding are not entirely clear. But we do know some of the factors that have resulted in such problems for women and babies.

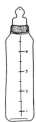

The Invention of Bottles
and Artificial Milks

Until the early twentieth century, substitutes for breastfeeding were not readily available for all women. Mothers who were well off could hire women to breastfeed in their place (wet nurses). Other mothers gave special substitutes of cow's or goat's milk, bread, and spices. The babies of these mothers died more often than those of mothers who breastfed.

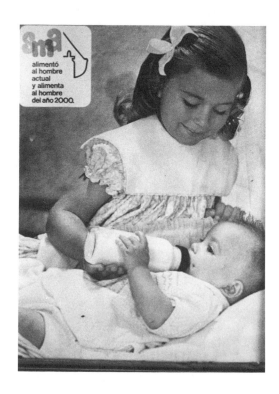

The invention of feeding bottles made artificial feeding more possible throughout the world. This Mexican poster shows how accepted bottle feeding has become in most countries.

Bottle feeding and breastfeeding are considered by many to be interchangeable and equal because bottle feeding is so heavily advertised and breastfeeding so misunderstood.

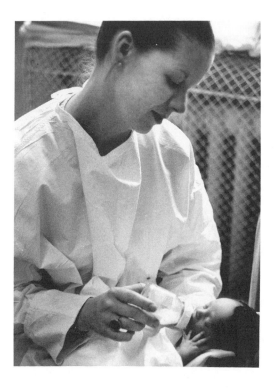

This is called "detached bottle feeding" because there is little body contact between the woman and the baby, as if the only important part of feeding were getting the food into the baby's stomach.

Commercial artificial formulas became available in the late nineteenth century. These were promoted by the manufacturers, and sometimes by the medical profession, as safe, even though they had never been tested on babies.

As the use of artificial substitutes for breast milk grew in Western culture, the knowledge about breastfeeding diminished. At the same time women started to work full days away from their babies, partly as a result of the World Wars, when women were needed to work in the factories, and partly because of the slowly increasing emancipation of women. No one really understood the impact this would have on child rearing.

Doctors then began to pay increasing attention to childbirth, and the results were mostly far from helpful. The advice written for mothers and caregivers by the new breed of infant feeding "experts" shows just how misguided much of this medical advice was. For example, breastfeeding mothers were taught to limit every breastfeed both in frequency and duration. Supplemental bottle feeding became widespread, probably because babies were left hungry after inadequate breastfeeds.

Modern Interventions in Birth and Infant Care

In the early 1900s widespread changes began to be introduced into the care of women at birth. Interventions in childbirth, many of them unnecessary, became routine. Gradually the hospital became the normal environment for birth. Interventions that were necessary in a few special situations quickly became the norm. Routine interventions included:

- Separating mothers and babies immediately after birth

- Placing healthy newborn babies in separate nurseries for observation

- Limiting the close contact between mothers and babies

- Scheduling and limiting breastfeeds

- Introducing bottles of artificial milk or sugar water to all breastfed babies

- Not allowing breastfeeding at night

- Teaching mothers to take the baby off the breast when the baby was judged to have had enough, usually after a specified time

- Encouraging the continued separation of mothers and babies at home, by advising parents to sleep in rooms separate from their babies' rooms right from birth

- Warning parents that picking babies up and cuddling them between feeds would spoil them

Bottles, schedules, and the separation of mothers and babies are interventions in breastfeeding, in just the same way as inductions, the use of oxytocin in labor, and cesarean sections are interventions in birth.

Just like all interventions in birth, they may be appropriate for a few .mothers and babies. But they all have harmful side effects that outweigh the benefits when routinely applied to the majority of mothers and babies. Because these interventions now happen so often, most people have come to accept them as normal, often not questioning their use.

A good example of an intervention in birth that most accept as normal is not permitting a woman to eat or drink in labor, instead using

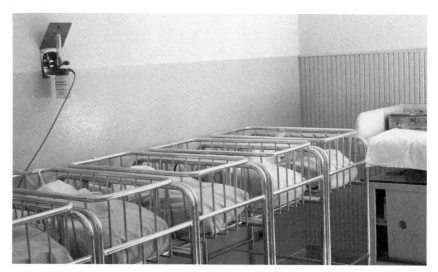

With routine intervention in normal birth has come the routine practice of separating babies from their mothers after birth. This is a hospital nursery in Italy, but it is typical now in many countries.

an intravenous (IV) drip, which is painful and restricts movement. This is similar to giving newborn babies bottles of sugar water (which has no nutritional value and actually causes hypoglycemia), rather than letting them breastfeed freely. It is easy to forget the harm that IVs and sugar water can do, and also to forget that women and babies need real nourishment in labor and afterward.

The use of breast milk substitutes and of interventions in birth and breastfeeding has now spread from Western countries to virtually all countries. Their impact is felt all over the world, even in countries where breastfeeding was, until very recently, the norm. There are still a few societies where breastfeeding is the normal way of feeding a baby. We have a lot to learn from mothers who breastfeed their babies without interventions.

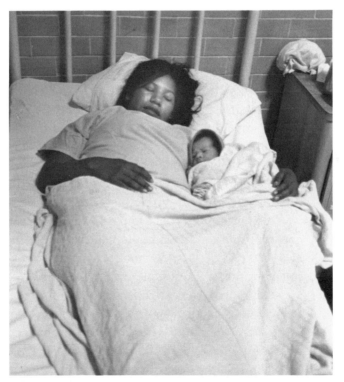

In most parts of the world mothers and newborn babies are kept together right from birth. This day-old Central American baby and her mother sleep together. If a mother prefers, she can place her baby in a little crib which is next to every mother's hospital bed.

The Separation of Women and Babies from Each Other and from Social Contact

Mothers and babies are often separated not just after birth, but also after they go home. Putting babies to sleep in rooms separate from those of their parents is one form of separation. Mothers leaving the home for a full working day is another.

Choosing whether to go right back to work is a dilemma many women face. In cultures in which home and work are separated and in which there is little social support for women who stay at home, women often must work outside the home and even outside the local community. Separation therefore lasts even longer than the working day. It is not unusual for a mother to travel an hour to and an hour from her work. Women need to work for many reasons: to earn money, for social contact, and to maintain promotion prospects in careers, which are shaped by the belief that workers (both women and men) should always put work first, never families or relationships.

In some countries (such as the United States and the United Kingdom) there is little support for women who wish to breastfeed and work outside the home. In other places, such as in Scandinavia, laws exist that enable women to work and have time and facilities to be with their babies and breastfeed during the work day.

A woman may choose to put her child in day care even if she does not work outside the home. In cultures in which the nuclear family is held as the ideal, it is sometimes hard for women to find enough adult company and support while caring for their own babies at home. Depression is now common among women in Western societies who stay at home to care for their babies and who become isolated from other adults. It is unhealthy to be separated from social support, especially when caring for young children. Some women assume that regular separation in this way means that they cannot continue to breastfeed. In fact they can, but they need support and facilities to do so, and these are not often available.

Working Away from Your Baby
(see also page 11)

Until societies that separate women and babies from other adults change, it will be necessary for some women to go out to work while they have very young babies, and to put young babies in full-time day care, in spite of the problems this causes. Many women find the demands of both breastfeeding and working outside the home too difficult, so they stop breastfeeding. Others find it hard to maintain their milk supply when separated, and find they have to stop even though they do not want to. The best ways to prepare for breastfeeding when you work outside the home are:

- Get breastfeeding off to a good start

- Prevent problems

- Learn early how to express milk

The Acceptance of Bottles as
the Normal Way of Feeding

Over the years most societies have become more comfortable with bottles than with breasts, partly because most people have bottle fed, and partly because of discomfort with the exposure of breasts. In several countries there is little experience of successful breastfeeding. And in most countries bottle feeding is seen as more normal than breastfeeding. Have you ever seen a breastfeeding mother on television? Have you ever seen breastfeeding mother and child dolls?

Think about how people often react with discomfort or criticism if a woman breastfeeds when outside her own home in Western countries. Breastfeeding is not an accepted part of modern life (although even up until World War II, it was common to see women in the United States and the United Kingdom breastfeeding in public). How would you feel if you were told you could not eat your dinner in public?

One of the most obvious symbols of the "normality" of bottle feeding is the common use of the bottle shape to indicate a feeding room in an airport or shopping center.

The acceptance of bottles is often unconscious. How many times have you heard people say things such as, "your breasts will be empty after feeding"? Breasts are never empty: they make milk all the time. Only bottles are empty after feeding.

A common question mothers ask is, "How can I know how much milk my baby is getting?" You do not need to know the exact amount. The common use of bottles has accustomed people in Western countries to seeing how much babies drink. Thus they feel uncomfortable if they do not see it and cannot measure it.

Look carefully at the advertising for baby products and even at the birth congratulations cards that you get. Many of these include baby bottles.

Breastfeeding has been forced to meet the standards of bottle feeding. This is the opposite of the way it should be: artificial feeding should be required to meet the standards of breastfeeding.

A Lost Confidence in Breastfeeding

The common use of bottles and lack of experience with breastfeeding helps to explain why so many women have no confidence in their own bodies or their own babies when breastfeeding. For example, women have been told that giving feeds at certain times is the best way to feed. In fact, if they listened to their babies rather than this unhelpful advice, they would feed when the baby was hungry, not when the clock read a certain time.

Feeding by schedule can also harm the mother. Her breasts become engorged because they are not milked efficiently, and this causes pain and tissue damage. A mother responding to her own body would feed her baby more often and thus prevent or alleviate the problem.

It is easy to see, however, why people have lost confidence in breastfeeding. Because so many women, including the mothers of many of today's mothers, have bottle fed, there is little experience of normal breastfeeding in their communities. Women who have breastfed have often had problems because of the lack of experience and support around them. Problems have become "normal."

The Problems for Health Workers

Remember that health workers are affected by cultural norms too. Whether they are nurses, midwives, doctors, lactation consultants, or nutritionists, they are not immune to societal beliefs and experiences. Bottle feeding has been accepted for several generations in some Western countries. Textbooks and teaching for health workers are full of inaccurate advice. Much of the teaching of health workers in developing countries too is based on the experiences and textbooks of Western medicine, in spite of the obvious lack of relevance of such information for most developing countries.

So health workers in most cultures find it hard to learn from experience or from books that give new information. They are used to the common interventions, such as timing feeds and giving bottles, often not understanding that it can be otherwise.

For health workers to be confident in caring for you, they need to have experience working with confident breastfeeding women. Because this is rare, they depend on the misinformation they have learned.

It is striking that no modern health care system that we know of has a rational approach to infant feeding. Every system around the world contains at least some practices that are both irrational and actually damaging to breastfeeding. These include the routine interventions that we talked about earlier, and the fact that care is concentrated around the time of birth, with virtually no care for the mother and baby after birth in some countries, particularly in the United States.

In the United States, for example, where women give birth in hospitals and go home a day or two after birth, it is rare for women to receive *any* professional care at home at all. Where does a woman who needs skilled care after birth turn to for help?

It is understandably difficult for health workers who have little experience with breastfeeding, who have a fund of misinformation from textbooks, and who are often not around when problems occur, to offer women the help they need. No wonder the most common solution offered to mothers with problems is "Try bottle feeding."

Mixed Messages

Many health workers and laypeople do know that breastfeeding should be different from the way it has been. They have heard of many of the helpful practices. But they often have too little experience to truly have confidence in these practices. This often results in people giving mixed messages to women.

These people may be genuinely supportive of breastfeeding, but may say something like, "Yes, demand feeding is best for your baby;

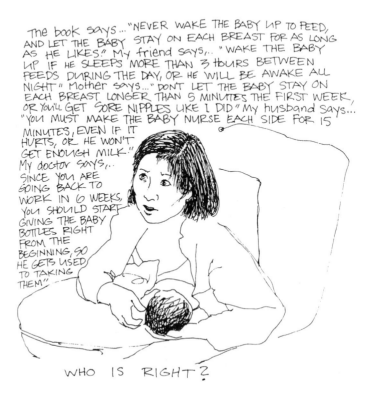

The book says..."NEVER WAKE THE BABY UP TO FEED, AND LET THE BABY STAY ON EACH BREAST FOR AS LONG AS HE LIKES." My friend says,.. "WAKE THE BABY UP IF HE SLEEPS MORE THAN 3 hours BETWEEN FEEDS DURING THE DAY, OR HE WILL BE AWAKE ALL NIGHT" Mother says..."DON'T LET THE BABY STAY ON EACH BREAST LONGER THAN 5 MINUTES THE FIRST WEEK, OR YOU'LL GET SORE NIPPLES LIKE I DID" My husband says... "YOU MUST MAKE THE BABY NURSE EACH SIDE FOR 15 MINUTES, EVEN IF IT HURTS, OR HE WON'T GET ENOUGH MILK." My doctor says,.. SINCE YOU ARE GOING BACK TO WORK IN 6 WEEKS, YOU SHOULD START GIVING THE BABY BOTTLES RIGHT FROM THE BEGINNING, SO HE GETS USED TO TAKING THEM."

WHO IS RIGHT?

There is so much said about breastfeeding.

you'll find that he'll probably want to feed every three to four hours or so." Such a statement may leave you wondering what is wrong when your baby sleeps for two hours or five hours between feeds.

Another example is, "Let the baby feed as long as she wants; I will show you how to take her off the breast when she has had enough." You may then wonder how you can tell when she has had enough, instead of realizing that she will let you know by coming off the breast herself.

Some of the strongest of these mixed messages come from the companies that manufacture artificial substitutes for human breast milk. Advertisements for artificial milk often carry a subtle (or sometimes obvious) message that artificial milk will be necessary when breastfeeding fails. That is why the World Health Organization has produced a code of practice for the marketing of artificial milks. The message advertisements often give is that breastfeeding will not work, even if it is better than substitutes. We call this the breast-is-best-*but* approach.

Although artificial milk companies have attempted to produce substances that babies can tolerate and thrive on, and although their products are useful in some circumstances, the dissemination of mixed messages is damaging and inaccurate.

We all need to learn to trust in the ability of women's bodies to breastfeed successfully. Instead of thinking, breast is best *but* . . . people need to believe the truth: breast *is* best.

But it is only possible for people to truly have this confidence by either personally experiencing successful breastfeeding or by seeing others do it.

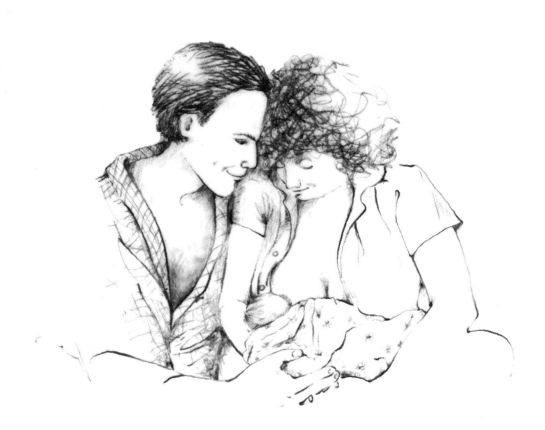

Things You Will Hear that Aren't True: Modern Myths

☆ *One of the problems you will have to cope with when you are breast-feeding, or planning to, is that many people will give you different, sometimes conflicting, advice and hints about feeding.*

We explained some of the reasons for this (see pages 158–159). In addition, many people who have breastfed (or have heard of others who have), or who have cared for breastfeeding women, will give you hints based on their experience.

These hints may be invaluable. Or they may be quite wrong. This is not because these friends or helpers *intend* to mislead you; it is because of confusion and lack of knowledge about breastfeeding.

This may be true of much of the advice given by health workers, family, and friends.

You will have to battle to disentangle fact from fantasy! We hope the information that follows will help.

MYTH: You must prepare your nipples in pregnancy to toughen them. If you do not they will become sore and damaged.

REALITY: Nipples do not need to be tough, because with the right position they will not get damaged or be subjected to any friction inside the baby's mouth (see page 60). No form of preparation has been shown to be of help in avoiding damage.

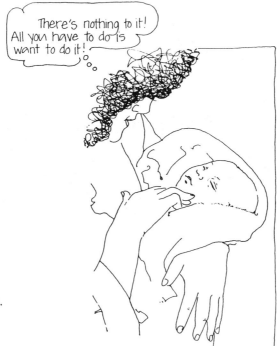

There's nothing to it! All you have to do is want to do it!

Some women think it's so easy, there's nothing to it.

MYTH: Women who have fair skin, red hair, or blue eyes will get sore nipples because they have delicate, easily damaged skin.

REALITY: No studies have ever shown that this is the case. These women, like all women, simply need to have help with positioning, so that their nipples do not get damaged (see pages 52–65).

MYTH: You must feed your baby immediately after birth or breastfeeding will not work.

REALITY: This has never been shown to be the case. It has, however, been shown that in cultures where immediate separation of mother and baby is the custom, women who feed within two hours of birth go on to breastfeed longer than those who do not.

There are other cultures where women do not breastfeed for the first two or three days, and during that time the baby is given other fluids or food instead of breast milk. These women still breastfeed successfully.

There is no critical period, no crucial time beyond which breastfeeding will not work. The ideal time to breastfeed is within the first couple of hours of birth (see page 31), but don't panic if you can't or if your baby doesn't want to yet. Remember that even mothers who have adopted babies have been able to stimulate their milk supply.

MYTH: You must time your baby's feeds, especially during the first few days, to prevent sore nipples.

REALITY: Sore nipples are caused by bad positioning, not by the amount of time your baby spends at the breast. In fact, limiting feeding time actually *causes* problems for babies (see page 79).

MYTH: Babies must feed from both breasts at every feed, or the milk supply will not be stimulated well enough.

REALITY: Babies should be allowed to decide what they want at each feed; any other method causes problems (see pages 76–79).

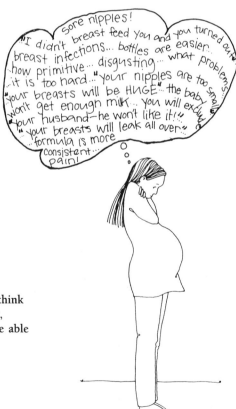

Some women think it's so difficult, they'll never be able to do it.

MYTH: Babies must feed from only one breast at each feed; that is all they need.

REALITY: This is the opposite of the preceding myth, but is equally popular. Again, babies should take what they need, not what rules and regulations decide is best (see page 79).

MYTH: You must drink lots of fluids (up to twelve to fourteen glasses a day) or you won't make enough milk.

REALITY: Studies show that this is not the case. All you need to do is drink when you are thirsty, rather than forcing yourself to drink more. Some women do get very thirsty, especially as they start to feed.

It is all right to drink whenever you want to. But be sure not to forget to drink; some women look after their babies more than themselves. If your urine is dark or strong-smelling, then you definitely need to drink more.

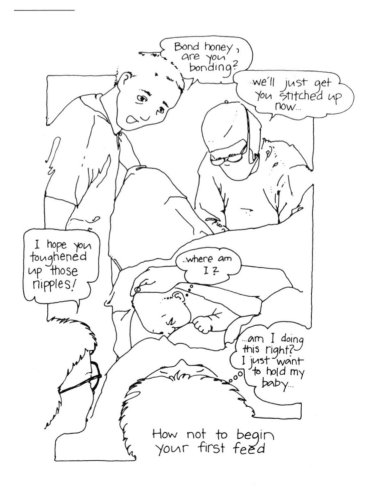

How not to begin your first feed.

How not to begin your first feed.

MYTH: Most breastfed babies need bottles of water or artificial milk or they won't get enough fluid.

REALITY: On the contrary, giving extra fluids to a breastfed baby can reduce your milk supply and interfere with the special properties of breast milk. The colostrum and milk that you produce is all your baby needs, as long as you are feeding without problems and not limiting feeding times (see page 79).

MYTH: The amount of milk a baby gets in a breastfeed is related to the length of that feed.

REALITY: Studies have shown that some babies feed for four minutes to get the same amount as other babies take in twenty-five minutes. Each baby has her own rate of feeding, and each woman has her own rate of milk release. You and your baby will work out your own pattern, as long as the positioning is correct.

MYTH: To help her nipples to heal, a mother with sore or bleeding nipples should:

- Rest her nipples,

- Use chlorhexidine gluconate 0.2 percent spray (Rotorsept),

- Use a nipple shield,

- Use a cream or lotion, or

- Stop breastfeeding

REALITY: Unless the mother solves the *cause* of the problem (which is always either a positioning difficulty, an infection, or a skin reaction), then nothing will help. Some of the treatments just listed may actually make her problem worse. None will fix it, unless stopping breastfeeding can be called fixing it (see pages 128–131).

MYTH: If you've fed before, you must know what you're doing.

REALITY: Each baby is different and you need to learn each time how to breastfeed *this* baby. Having done it before helps, but it is not a guarantee. You can still have problems.

MYTH:	Flexible, or demand, feeding is harder on the mother.
REALITY:	Feeding your baby whenever she wants is the best thing to keep her contented. If you don't do this, then she will cry more than she needs, and this will disturb you and your whole family. This is *not* easier on the mother (see page 79).

MYTH:	If your baby feeds only from the breast, you will never get enough sleep at night.
REALITY:	It is true that breastfed babies wake in the night more often than bottle fed babies. And it is true that lack of sleep is the hardest problem for parents of young children. Unlike bottle feeding, however, once you and your baby are breastfeeding well, you do not have to be fully awake during a feed. Have your baby sleep near you, take him into bed when he cries (or have him sleep in the same bed with you and skip this step), feed lying on your side, and fall back to sleep (see page 40).

MYTH:	Women with engorged breasts should not express milk to relieve them.
REALITY:	Gentle expression of a little milk helps relieve engorgement and swelling (edema). It does *not* make it worse (see pages 123–124).

MYTH:	Young babies always cry a lot, so you should leave your baby to cry.
REALITY:	A baby has all the feelings an adult has. She cries because she has a need. Crying only expresses pain or upset, nothing else. People comfort adults who cry. A baby cannot meet most of her own needs, and she needs us to take her crying seriously; she needs comfort too (see pages 137–144).

MYTH:	If you and your baby have serious breastfeeding problems, don't expect to be able to continue to breastfeed.
REALITY:	Most breastfeeding problems can be fixed, even quite serious ones. Often the solution is simple and improvement happens quickly. The sooner you try to deal with your problem, the easier it is. Don't wait until it grows; deal with it now. See page 121 for a listing of problems and solutions.

MYTH:	Orthodontic bottle or pacifier teats are the teats most similar to mothers' nipples.
REALITY:	Orthodontic teats are firm and hold a definite shape. They are not soft, responsive, or stretchy like mothers' nipples. We still do not know what shape of teat is least harmful to the development of the baby's face.

MYTH: Your baby is sure to be feeding well if he has six to eight wet diapers or nappies a day.

REALITY: In assessing your baby's health, you need to judge several different factors, not just one. (For a listing, see page 87.)

MYTH: You must begin to give solid foods when your baby is four months old or she will be nutritionally deprived.

REALITY: Babies who are breastfeeding well can breastfeed without any other food for at least six months, and some for longer. What matters is that they are content and continue to grow well.

MYTH: You must stop breastfeeding by nine months, or you will never get the baby to stop.

REALITY: This is not true. You and your baby can work out the best time for you both to cut down and then stop breastfeeding.

          There are no hard and fast rules, and it will not harm your baby to continue for a long while, even after you have introduced other foods, if you both want to do so. In many cultures children are normally breastfed for three or four years.

MYTH: You must feed only from the breast until the baby wants to stop, or you will harm her psychologically.

REALITY: This myth is the opposite of the preceding myth. You feel pressure to continue longer than you may want to. You and your baby should work out together what is best for you both. As is true in any good relationship, you may both need to compromise.

MYTH: You will spoil your baby if you give him what he wants whenever he wants it.

REALITY: Responding to babies' needs is not the same as spoiling them. Babies need to be fed when they are hungry, to sleep when they are tired, to be cuddled when they feel lonely, and to be comforted when they are sad. This will result in contented babies, not little dictators. A contented baby is better equipped to handle the normal pains and frustrations that are part of being human than is a baby who is often frustrated and upset, but rarely comforted.

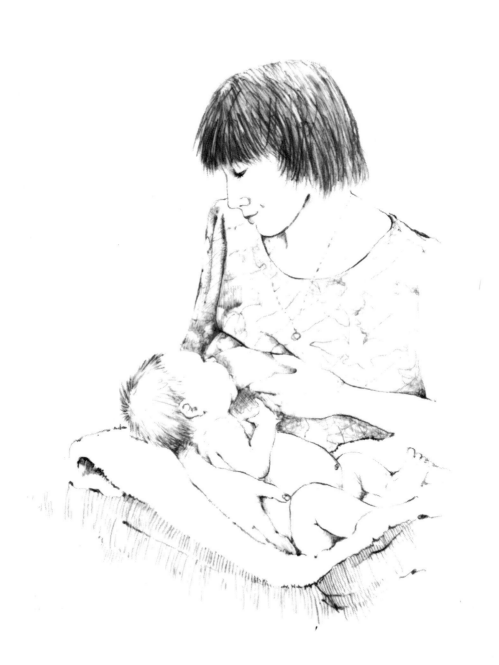

Women's Breastfeeding Stories: Case Studies

Every breastfeeding experience is different, and each mother faces different circumstances and challenges.

Some women have good support; others have none. Some have babies who feed well and easily from the start; others struggle for a while. Some produce lots of milk; others produce less. Some mothers are able to stay home full time while their babies are young; some must go back to work and leave their babies in the care of others for many hours a day.

Dealing with your own circumstances means that you need to understand the basic principles we outline in this book, and then adapt them to yourself and your family. To show the wide variety of situations that women face when they breastfeed, we have included stories about women from different countries and ethnic backgrounds, showing how each woman dealt with her breastfeeding problem.

All of the women in these stories are people with whom we ourselves have worked. We've chosen problematic stories rather than easy ones to give you confidence in your own ability to work things out.

BECKY'S STORY: *A Sleepy Baby Who Was Losing Weight*

Jonathan was Becky's first baby, and she really wanted to breastfeed him. Her birth took place in a hospital. She had an epidural anesthetic during her labor, but went on to have a normal spontaneous delivery with a small episiotomy.

She kept Jonathan with her after the birth and fed him as soon as they were settled into bed together. A maternity nurse helped her with the first feed. Becky went home on the second day without anyone at the hospital watching her feed again or realizing that she had a problem. But Becky knew.

At home she got really discouraged when, after trying to put Jonathan on her breast as well as she could at each feed, he would cry fiercely and then get tired and lie there with her nipple in his mouth and fall back asleep. He was a normal-sized baby at birth (7½ pounds), but was down to 7 pounds after a week. Becky became even more frustrated when she found that when she gave him a bottle, he would drink thirstily and go to sleep contented. The swollen breasts that she had on the third and fourth days after birth made her problems even worse. She became so sore that she found it even harder to put her baby on her breast.

Becky asked for help from many people. By nine days after birth, she had seen five health workers. All tried to help; each gave different advice. She was told to wake Jonathan every two hours and try to feed because he was still losing weight. She was also advised to give him three bottles of artificial milk a day.

Jonathan and his mother had never had even one good, pleasurable breastfeed. In spite of the fact that Jonathan was not even feeding very often, Becky had developed tender nipples. Giving up breastfeeding seemed to be the only solution. She was worried about her baby's weight, felt frustrated at every feed, and was exhausted from getting up every two hours to wake and feed him. One pediatrician watched her feed and checked her positioning, but noticed that although Jonathan appeared to go on to the breast well, he gave a few weak sucks and stopped. The pediatrician could think of no reason for the baby's seeming disinterest, and brought Jonathan to see us.

We saw Becky nine days after the birth. Her pediatrician came with her to see what she could learn, so she could help other women with Becky's problem. We first watched Becky try to begin a feed. There were two problems with the way she was feeding Jonathan. One was that she was concentrating so hard on his positioning that she didn't think of her own. She chose to sit in a high-backed rocking chair, which was similar to the one she used at home. In this chair she leaned backward, and that pulled her breasts away from her baby. The other difficulty was that, although the position of the baby's mouth on her breast looked fairly good, his body was not tucked close

enough into hers. The combination of these two problems, neither of them seemingly serious, had resulted in Jonathan not being able to take quite enough of her breast into his mouth, no matter how hard he tried.

Once Becky sat upright, with enough pillows to support her back and her baby's body as he lay on her lap, and once she held Jonathan tucked close into her, the change in his behavior was immediate! Instead of taking a few weak sucks and falling asleep or crying with frustration, he started to feed strongly and well. "It doesn't hurt at all!" Becky said, surprised. Jonathan fed for twenty-five minutes on one side and then let go of the breast. She sat him up for a minute to burp, and then she positioned him on her other breast. She wanted to learn to breastfeed lying on her side so we showed her how to do this. He took the second side just as well and let go when done. He fell asleep, full and contented.

Becky felt for the first time the joy of a problem-free, pain-free feed. After help to have one good feed, and an understanding of what had caused her problems, she went on to breastfeed her son well and with enjoyment. A week later Jonathan had gained half a pound in weight and this improvement continued.

Becky had difficulty in positioning Jonathan at her breast partly because she did not have good help in the early days after birth, but also because Jonathan was a sleepy baby, possibly because of the medication used during his birth. It is often the case that with sleepy babies the positioning has to be absolutely right, a small difference can prevent them from feeding.

If the nipple is not in just the right place in the baby's mouth, the baby may not get the signals he needs. If he is put to the breast regularly, but is unable to feed well, he soon gets frustrated and cries, and then falls asleep while feeding, with the nipple still in his mouth. This can become an impossible situation for both mother and baby. If not solved quickly, it can lead to a decision to bottle feed. It is easy to understand why.

Sore Nipples, Early Supplementing, and Return to Work with a Very Young Baby

Meili was a mother of a six-year-old, expecting her next baby. She had had problems feeding Lily, her first. Lily had been eight weeks' premature, had been delivered by cesarean, and had spent six weeks in the special care nursery. Meili had used a breast pump at first to get her milk supply going, and Lily had been given her mother's milk; but when Meili had started to breastfeed Lily, she had developed sore nipples that had quickly become badly damaged and bled. She had stopped breastfeeding and gone back to using the breast pump, feeding Lily her breast milk from the bottle. After a week or two, she had stopped pumping too. "My milk just went," she told us. "I couldn't get any out."

In preparation for their second baby, Meili and her husband, Chin, went to childbirth classes. They wanted to have a normal delivery this time. They also read a lot about breastfeeding. They arranged to use the money Meili had saved from her job to hire a full-time housekeeper for the first two weeks. Chin planned time off from work to be at home for the first ten days, so that together they could get the feeding right.

Meili went into labor at term with this child, but after nine hours the baby was found to be in a breech position. Meili was put on an intravenous drip in labor, and not allowed to drink anything. Meili was given a cesarean section with a spinal anesthetic (cesarean sections are often done today simply because the baby is breech, despite the fact that breech babies can often be safely delivered vaginally). After the cesarean she was given only ice chips to suck for the first two days. Meili was dehydrated and felt unwell for the first two days after the birth; she had a temperature and a sore throat. In spite of this difficult and disappointing beginning, Meili put her new baby, Peiwin, to her breast soon after birth and breastfed her. She fed lying down, as this was the most comfortable position for her after her surgery.

From the second day on, Meili had sore nipples. Her husband, who had been told that to stimulate the milk supply a woman needs to breastfeed for at least fifteen minutes on each side, prompted her to keep feeding even though it hurt, and he timed each feed. Meili's nipples quickly became damaged and bled. By day four she had stopped breastfeeding, and had gone back to the pumping and bottle feeding she had used with her first child. When we saw them at home nine days after birth, both Meili and Chin expressed great disappointment that breastfeeding didn't work.

Meili's cesarean scar was healing well and her nipples were nearly healed. She was giving Peiwin bottles at every feed, alternating artificial milk with her breast milk, which she expressed by a hand pump. She supplemented with artificial milk, we learned, because Chin felt that perhaps she wasn't producing enough milk to feed the baby. The baby fed every two to three hours, and it was obvious that both parents were working hard to give her the best they could.

After we watched Meili put her baby on her breast, it was clear to us why she was having problems with her nipples. She sat in a comfortable chair to feed, but she was tense and bent forward over the baby, who lay on a pillow in her lap. Peiwin was not held close enough to her mother's body, and she lay more on her back than on her side. This meant that she had to turn her head to find the breast. In addition, she didn't take enough breast in her mouth.

The baby was patient as Meili settled herself to feed. She went on the breast eagerly, but with her mouth not wide open enough, so her gums were fixed tightly over the nipple. Because Meili had large nipples and her baby had a small mouth (not an unusual combination for

Asian mothers and babies), it was easy for Peiwin to take the nipple rather than the breast. Meili also was in the habit of keeping a finger on her breast, next to the areola, to keep the baby's nose clear. This tended to pull the breast back out of the baby's mouth. To compound the problems, Chin gave a constant stream of instructions as she fed.

Only small, but important, changes were needed with what Meili was doing. First, she needed to sit more upright. Second, she needed to hold Peiwin's body facing hers and closer to her own. Third, she needed to brush Peiwin's lips with her nipple, wait for Peiwin's mouth to gape open wide, and then move the baby onto her breast.

Once she had these things described to her, Meili changed her position and tried to move Peiwin's open mouth onto her breast. She tried several times before getting it right. Then, for the first time, Peiwin drew Meili's nipple well back into her mouth and began to feed strongly and deeply. "It doesn't hurt at all!" Meili exclaimed, not quite believing it. As her baby continued to feed, she noted that although her nipple felt "funny"—as if it was being stretched—there was no pain. When her baby came off the breast, Meili noted with obvious delight that her nipple was not squashed flat, as it had been after all her other feeds, but was quite round.

"It was so nearly right, but not quite!" observed Chin, who had watched carefully. They both had explanations for why other helpers had not been able to fix the problem. Meili said, "The difference was that they did it for me! I was not even involved. They put her on and then left me to it. It helped to have your hand right over mine, guiding it—and then for you to watch me do it myself." Chin noted that the problem with breastfeeding books was that it was not possible to work out their particular problem from looking at a tiny diagram. "We needed a photograph of how it should be,

along with a drawing, and a picture of what it looked like if it was wrong."

This was a classic case of how feeding could be almost right, but not quite, thereby ending up all wrong. A number of details were just a bit wrong: the mother's body position, the baby's body position, and the baby's mouth position on the breast. Together it added up to damaged nipples, a baby not getting the right balance of milk, the breasts not making enough milk, and a husband who had lost confidence in his wife's ability to breastfeed their baby. Added to this was the combination of a mother who was disappointed about having a possibly unnecessary repeat cesarean, a mother with large nipples, and a baby with a small mouth. The well-meaning but anxious concern of her husband made Meili nervous, and she had lost self-confidence.

We left their home after two hours, with Peiwin having had a good feed from both breasts (her first ever) and then having dropped off the breast after she was done, much to her mother's surprise. It had taken a few attempts by Meili to get her baby on right. We were careful to tell them both that it would take practice and a number of attempts before it would be quite right. There might well be one or two feeds where she wouldn't be able to get it right at all. But it would gradually get better as she and her baby learned. "Don't worry," we said. "You have the principles right. You just need practice. Be patient, both of you."

We encouraged them not to have Meili pump her milk or supplement with artificial milk for the next few days. We told them to expect Peiwin to feed often, around the clock, for a few days, while she and her mother's milk supply caught up with each other. We encouraged them to call us if they needed help, but Meili and Chin assured us that they would now manage by themselves.

A week later, when we checked by phone to see how Meili was doing, disappointment was in her voice as she said she was back to pumping and bottle feeding. She had had several good breastfeeds the day after we had seen her, but her nipples had become slightly sore as she had practiced getting her baby on right, and sometimes it hadn't worked. She had lost her confidence again, and even those good breastfeeds hadn't restored it. Chin had told her she should have toughened her nipples before the birth.

It seemed that Chin's concern, added to her lack of confidence (partly resulting from her feelings about her cesarean and partly from her first nine days of problematic feeding) made her unsure of her ability to breastfeed successfully. We offered again to come and sit with her for a feed and to observe and help her, or to find someone else who could come each day for a while, just to be a support while she practiced. She sounded delighted to hear that we were confident that she could get the baby back on the breast again, but she declined our offer to visit. Chin was still off work and it seemed he preferred to be her sole support. Because he was going to go back to work the next day, we suggested that Meili do her breastfeeding while she was alone, and supplement only while he was home, because his feeling that Peiwin was not getting enough milk led him to push Meili to supplement.

Meili agreed. She said she would like it if we would call her once in a while to see how she was doing. One of us called five days later and Meili said, "I've just lost all my confidence!" She had given up trying to breastfeed. The one day she had done it, the baby had gone on wrong once and within several strong sucks she had felt pain, so she hadn't tried again that feed. She had tried the next day, but Peiwin hadn't seemed interested in her breast, so she had given up.

Meili was still expressing milk, feeding Peiwin exclusively on her breast milk. But she had just been to see the pediatrician, who had told her that she was not giving her baby enough milk. "I just can't get more than 3½ ounces from the pump," she said with great

concern. We reminded her of how supplementing ended up decreasing her milk supply. We suggested that she continue to express milk often and try once again to breastfeed, but only when there was no one else in the house, because she did best when no one made her anxious. The baby, we said, would have to relearn to take the breast; it would just take time and patience, and care in getting her on right.

Meili did not continue to breastfeed, but she remained dedicated in her efforts to give Peiwin her milk. At one month Peiwin was growing well and was a contented baby. She fed from a bottle, having breast milk for all but one feed. Meili and Chin had worked out a creative solution between them that was satisfactory to Meili. She would express regularly during the day, beginning at 8:00 A.M. From the time Chin got home from work he would take over feeding Peiwin, and at the same time Meili would sit with them and express her milk for the next feed. She would express milk up until the 11:00 P.M. feed, and then have to get up only once more in the night to express milk. Chin got up with her at that time and fed Peiwin, and at 5:00 A.M., when Peiwin awoke for another feed, he would let Meili sleep and feed the baby a bottle of artificial milk. This arrangement worked for everyone, and it continued to work well for almost two more months, but then the demands upon Meili increased.

Meili had known that she would have to return to work only ten weeks after the birth because that was all the paid maternity leave granted by her company. There were no provisions for on-site day care, and employees were not permitted to work flexible hours to enable them to take time off during the middle of the day to go and breastfeed. Meili had planned to continue feeding Peiwin her breast milk; throughout the day she would use a pump to express milk and then refrigerate it. When it came time to make preparations to return to her job, however, Meili reassessed her choices and decided to wean Peiwin. Although her workplace is only a few miles from home, working meant she would leave the house at 8:00 A.M. and not return until after 5:30 P.M. Because of her position as accounting manager, Meili knew that she would have much work to catch up on and that she could not realistically plan to express milk while at work.

Meili wanted to make the transition as easy as possible for Peiwin and herself. She had carefully arranged that the day care person would be the same woman who had helped at the house part-time since Peiwin's birth. Meili decided that Peiwin would spend the day at the baby-sitter's house, which was nearby. This woman had two children of her own in high school and was very comfortable with young babies, especially Peiwin, whose needs she knew well by the time Meili returned to work. The baby-sitter had only one other child to care for, an eighteen-month-old boy, so Peiwin would have a great deal of cuddling and individual attention. To avoid painful engorgement from stopping breastfeeding suddenly, Meili weaned Peiwin onto formula over several weeks. The adjustment went well for both Peiwin and her mother, in part because Meili was comfortable with her child care arrangements and didn't feel guilty or anxious.

At her six-month checkup, Peiwin was pronounced strong, healthy, and big for a Chinese baby, which pleased her mother and father. She smiles easily and is good natured. She started sleeping through the night at six weeks, which made it much easier for Meili to return to work. To help Peiwin sleep, Meili and Chin tried to make sure that she had a large feed before bedtime. Each evening, after one of them bathed her, Peiwin would take a bottle of Meili's milk, but she would usually fall asleep after taking only a couple of ounces. Chin found that if he lay her down on her back, a position she usually didn't like, she would wake herself, and then he could feed her the rest of the bottle. This strategy worked, and she

continues to go to sleep without a lot of fussing, sometimes after talking to herself in her crib.

Meili combined traditional cultural advice and practices with modern assistance to make feeding work. She had worried that her breasts might not get enough stimulation from expressing milk to meet Peiwin's needs. She listened to her mother's advice and followed the ritual women in her ancestry had followed to assure an ample milk supply: "I made soup each day. Usually it was either a whole fish cooked in water with ginger and green onions, or pigs' knuckles cooked in water with peanuts. Otherwise I made chicken soup. I had these every day." Meili is not sure whether the soup made a difference, but she felt comfortable following the traditional advice and is glad that she did. "I really tried very hard. It took a lot of work."

Meili wondered why breastfeeding had been so difficult for her. We suggested that it was not any one factor, but a number of things that added up to a considerable problem. We reminded her how well she had done in the face of adversity, and she agreed; she is proud of her daughter and should take credit for how resourceful she and Chin have been. Meili told us that if they have a third child she will definitely get help from the beginning to ensure she starts out right. "Then I think I will probably be able to breastfeed all the time," she said.

JUDY'S STORY:
Too Much Milk

Three years after giving up breastfeeding her baby in frustration, Judy was still feeling the disappointment. It is never possible to diagnose problems in retrospect, but Judy wanted to talk to us about what had happened to her, in order to gain some understanding of what had gone wrong. She hoped to have another baby, and very much wanted to breast-feed well. Judy had started leaking colostrum when she had been five months' pregnant, and had continued throughout her pregnancy. Her pregnancy had gone well and she had looked forward to birth.

She had had a normal labor, at term, and she had enjoyed giving birth. She told us proudly that she had pushed her daughter out in just thirty minutes. Clearly the birth had been a positive experience for Judy, unlike breast-feeding. The problems had begun when, after birth, the hospital staff had taken her baby, Jilly, to the nursery. Jilly had been hypo-glycemic and without asking Judy's permission the staff had tried to insert an intravenous line into the baby to give her some glucose. When Jilly had been brought to Judy two hours later, her head was shaved and there were several punctures where someone had tried to insert the needle. "Why didn't they just let me feed her in the first place?" said Judy. "I had so much milk!" A nurse had helped her get breast-feeding started, and she had left the hospital without any idea that she would have problems at home.

Jilly had then gone onto the breast and had fed well from the start. Judy had had no nipple problems, and Jilly had sucked strongly and effectively. She had awakened every two hours to feed, fed for fifteen to twenty minutes, and then gone to sleep. She had never wanted the second breast. She had grown quickly. By only three days after birth she had gained al-most a pound, an unusual occurrence.

Judy's abundant milk supply had contin-ued. One week after birth, Jilly had started to spit up some of every feed. A week later six of Judy's relatives, including her mother-in-law, had come to stay for two weeks. It had been Christmas, and Judy's in-laws had wanted to spend it with the new baby. This had caused problems for Judy and Dan, who had felt they had to look after their houseful of guests. Judy had become very tired, especially as Jilly still had been feeding every two hours.

At three weeks after birth, Judy had no-ticed her breasts were very full and heavy at each feed. She had started having to express milk before every feed, just so Jilly could take her breast. She remembered saying to her baby, "Please feed so my breasts won't hurt!" When she had been feeding, she had leaked so much from the opposite breast that she had had to hold a cup under the other breast or she would get soaked with milk.

Jilly had continued to bring up milk after each feed. At one month she had had two epi-sodes of severe projectile vomiting. Because they did not happen again, and because Jilly had continued to gain one pound a week, Judy had continued to feed. By this time Jilly had often pulled off the breast and choked or gag-ged while feeding. It had looked to Judy as if she was getting too much milk too fast. By this stage Judy had been always tired, unable to sit back and enjoy feeds because of her full breasts, the leaking milk, and Jilly's choking and spitting up. She had turned to local breast-feeding counselors and health care practitioners for help, but no one had been able to tell her why she had so much milk.

All this time Jilly had been well and gain-ing weight fast—too fast for Judy's comfort. She had been a happy baby. Her stools had been quite normal, soft and yellow. Judy had gone back to work at ten weeks, and had expressed milk each day for her baby. Expression had been easy because she had had so much. The problem had been that it was hard to stay away from Jilly for any length of time, because Judy would quickly get full and sore.

Judy had breastfed for only three months, but, she said, "It felt like a year." Her life had been dominated by feeding and milk. With great regret she had put Jilly on a bottle and formula milk.

It is always hard to diagnose problems in ret-rospect, but there are important clues in this story that point to Judy's simply having had too much breast milk. It had probably not been a problem of balancing the foremilk and hind-milk, because Jilly had always gone on well, finished the first breast first, and come off on her own. Also Jilly had had a normal stool, not the liquid, greenish stools that often indicate too much foremilk. It was not likely that it had been a positioning problem either. Judy had never had sore nipples or mastitis or any other indications of positioning difficulty. The baby had always taken her feeds in a reasonable length of time. Neither did it seem that it had been a letdown problem, because Judy had often found her breasts full, heavy, and leaking.

A very small number of women do produce too much breast milk. The first thing to do is to make sure that this really is the problem by ruling out the other causes. Often the problem resolves over two or three weeks. If not, then deliberately feeding from only one breast at each feed will limit breast stimulation and therefore milk supply. If all else fails, some women collect the excess milk and send it to the local milk bank.

KAREN'S STORY:
Constant Feeding but a Slow-Gaining Baby, Mastitis, and a Diagnosis of Milk Intolerance

Karen breastfed her first baby for ten months, in spite of having a range of problems, which included three episodes of mastitis. Her baby slept poorly at night and fed frequently, round the clock.

With Mark, her second baby, she hoped that breastfeeding would be easier, so that she could enjoy her baby, rather than being constantly tired. She had a standard hospital birth, with a vaginal delivery but numerous routine interventions in labor. She started breastfeeding soon after birth, but found the first two feeds especially difficult, and received little help from the hospital staff. She developed sore nipples within the first week, but she did have occasional good, pain-free feeds. More often than not, however, she found feeding painful. "If only I had a good midwife to help me!" she said.

Karen's nipples healed enough that she was able to continue to breastfeed, but she rarely had a pain-free feed. Mark was not a contented baby. At thirteen weeks after birth, when we first saw them, he was almost a "failure-to-thrive" baby. He wanted to feed every hour, had green, liquid stools, and his weight gain was well below normal. Because of this he had a little, pinched face.

When we watched Karen feeding, it became clear that there was a positioning difficulty. She held Mark's body close to hers, and she waited for his mouth to open wide. But she bent over him, tense, with her shoulders hunched and chest curled inward, so that her breasts hung straight down toward her baby. Then, as she moved him onto her breast, she bent the wrist of the hand supporting his head (Chloe calls this movement the flip), which bent his neck (it should be in a straight line with the back). This resulted in his chin dropping down toward his chest, a position that makes it almost impossible for a baby to feed well. It also buried Mark's nose in the breast, so Karen found she had to hold her breast out of the way so Mark could breathe.

Karen needed to learn to sit with her back erect (neither leaning back nor curled forward), and then to help Mark to take the breast straight on, rather than bending his neck inward as she put him on. She found it helped for her to support her breast, which slightly shaped her nipple so that Mark could take the breast more easily (see page 50). She was able to relax into the feed because there was no pain at all. Mark fed well, with deep, long suckles, unlike the way he had been doing for the past three months. Mark came off the breast when he was done, looking sated, and Karen was greatly relieved.

With a new understanding of the basic principles of breastfeeding, Karen felt confident enough to go back home and continue on her own. She was delighted to discover that feeding did not hurt at all. Nor did she any longer need to hold her breast away from Mark's nose. We heard from her a week later that Mark's behavior had changed dramatically with that first good feed. He had slept soundly on the drive home and had fed well the rest of the day. He was sleeping well between each feed and beginning to feed less at night. He was gaining weight rapidly.

Karen told us during her visit how she had learned about breastfeeding. She said that in her own career as a nurse, she had seen only problematic breastfeeding—never good, confident breastfeeding. She had seen bottle feeding, and she had a sense that what she had been doing was bottle feeding her baby with her breast. This meant that she had tried to put her breast into his mouth, rather than helping him to actively take her breast. She noted, "It's so easy to lose your confidence, even if you've done it wrong only once!"

She also talked about how problems with breastfeeding greatly affected the way women felt about breastfeeding. "So many of my friends want to breastfeed, but they've had problems with their first baby, and they just don't want to try it again." Karen believed it was important for women to have one-to-one skilled help when they need it, rather than just having the techniques shown to them and then being left on their own. She said it meant a lot to her that we had not done it for her, but had watched her body and her hands, had told her how to move them, and then had explained what had been right and what had been wrong with what she had tried.

We talked to Karen again when Mark was just over fifteen months old. She had continued breastfeeding him for nine months, at which time he gradually weaned himself. Over a few weeks, he cut down from six feeds a day to just one at night, and then to one every two or three nights until he stopped completely.

When we asked about problems Karen had while breastfeeding, an interesting story emerged. She had had three episodes of mastitis, the first one starting when Mark was about five months old. "And I'm sure it wasn't a problem with positioning," she told us. "That problem was solved, but I still got mastitis." She was given antibiotics on two of the three occasions, but she also breastfed as often as she could. "I knew that the best treatment was to feed," she said. "It just felt like there was a blockage, and all we had to do was clear it."

The pattern of Mark's weight gain remained the same throughout the time he was breastfed, slow but steady. He was happy and healthy, and Karen received nothing but encouragement from the health workers. Her health visitor was especially supportive and kept in close contact. Karen was never advised by her health professionals to supplement her breast milk with artificial milk or to stop breastfeeding, but Mark was watched carefully. Only two people suggested giving Mark extra bottles. One was Karen's mother-in-law who had had an identical problem breastfeeding one of her children and who dealt with it by feeding from both the breast and the bottle. The other person was her husband who was worried about Mark's slow weight gain. Karen told us she suspected that he wanted a chance to feed the baby a bottle himself. When he did try, Mark refused it. "I would have given up breastfeeding if I had been advised to do that by my doctor or health visitor," she said. "But because they supported me, I did what I really wanted to do and kept feeding."

As soon as Karen started to introduce other foods, a new problem emerged. Mark simply refused to take milk products, so she gave him solids, juice, and water. She occasionally tried to give him formula milk after she stopped breastfeeding but did not force him to take it, and he consistently refused. She had the same result when she tried giving Mark ordinary cow's milk when he was a year old. At about fourteen months, Karen discovered that Mark would take a yogurt-based fruit drink. Soon after drinking it, however, he developed severe eczema, and an intolerance to cow's milk was diagnosed.

An intolerance to cow's milk explains the symptoms that Karen and Mark had experienced. The combination of baby with slow weight gain in spite of efficient feeding and a mother with recurrent mastitis can indicate that the baby is intolerant to milk products. And a baby's refusal to take milk also points toward the baby's possible intolerance. In this case, a baby can be more perceptive than an adult.

As we talked with Karen, it became clear that both she and her husband have difficulty with milk products. Karen has eczema and her husband refuses all dairy products. Their older child, who had almost the same difficulties while breastfeeding as Mark, is allergic to a number of foods, including eggs.

Karen told us her only real concern after the diagnosis was Mark's calcium intake. But recently he has started to drink soy-based milk with no ill effects; since it contains calcium, she is no longer worried.

"But I do wonder about breastfeeding another child if we have one," she said. Karen's doctor advised her not to breastfeed another baby, partly because she had found a lump in her breast, which felt somewhat like mastitis, two months after she stopped breastfeeding Mark. This gradually disappeared over about six weeks. Her doctor was concerned about the amount of mastitis she had experienced and suggested that she bottle feed if she has more children. Bottle feeding would be a problem, however, if the next baby was milk intolerant too, and there would be concern about what to feed him or her.

We suggested that with her next baby, she exclude all dairy products from her own diet. Since this is difficult to do, we told her to talk with her health visitor and a nutritionist. A baby can be intolerant of dairy products passed over in the breast milk, and the only way to solve this problem is to remove them entirely from the mother's diet.

Karen faced a difficult challenge breastfeeding her baby, and she dealt with it remarkably well. With good support from her health workers, she continued to breastfeed as long as her baby wanted. She did not force Mark to drink milk he did not want and, when the intolerance was diagnosed, made sure that he got a balanced diet. Although she was disappointed that breastfeeding was more difficult than she had imagined, she was aware that Mark would have had difficulty with milk substitutes. "I know it was the best thing to do, and I'm glad we succeeded," she said. "I just hope it's not so hard the next time."

JENNY'S STORY:
Getting It Right with the Third Baby, but Facing a New Challenge — Breastfeeding a Critically Ill Baby

Jenny talked to us about her experience with Robbie, her nine-day-old son. She had been worried about breastfeeding, because she had had problems in the early days with Hugh and Tom, her first two children, who were now seven and three.

When she had had her first two babies, Jenny and her husband had been living in a part of the country where it was considered rude to breastfeed in public, or even to do it in front of guests in your own home. Jenny told us, "I always had to wait until visitors had gone or take the baby into another room." She had found this meant that she couldn't breastfeed when she and her baby needed to, and with each baby she had developed severe, painful engorgement a few days after birth. She also had had sore nipples for a few days.

This third time was different. They had moved across the country to a community where breastfeeding was seen as a normal and natural way of feeding babies, and people were not shocked when a woman fed in public. Ever since the influx of young, progressive-minded people in the late 1960s, Santa Cruz—a college town on the coast in Northern California—has been a community where breastfeeding is an ordinary part of life.

Jenny started breastfeeding Robbie, who weighed 8 pounds, 6 ounces at birth, shortly after he was born. She fed whenever he and she wanted to, whether she had visitors or was alone. She had no engorgement at all. She also said that she understood, without instruction, more about good positioning, as this was her third baby. Breastfeeding went smoothly and she never had sore nipples.

In Santa Cruz it is becoming common for women to spend the first month after birth at home, rather than moving right back into a busy life. This is a tradition in many cultures across the world, and helps to keep the world at bay. It honors a woman's need to have quiet time with her baby so she can recuperate and adjust to her new life. Jenny and Dave had decided during Jenny's pregnancy with Robbie to spend the first month of their new baby's life as quietly as possible. Jenny did not go out of the house at all for twenty-eight days, and Dave went out only to work and shop. Jenny said, "It's been wonderful: so relaxed and quiet."

Both Jenny and Dave commented to us that because their lives were usually so busy—with working, shopping, visiting, going out in the car, taking the older children out—it was hard to get the rest and time with a new baby that they and the baby needed. For Jenny and Dave, the way to deal with this was to cut down on anything that they did not have to do.

They certainly looked relaxed and breastfeeding was going fine without any outside help.

Jenny had noticed that from birth Robbie breathed somewhat faster than had her other babies. She had pointed this out to the midwife and a pediatrician and had been told that his breathing was within the normal range and, since his color was good and he was obviously thriving, there was no need for alarm. When Robbie was four months old, Jenny took him in for immunizations. At that time, the physician said he wanted to make sure Robbie's lungs were clear and suggested a chest x-ray. It was possible that Robbie had a minor form of bronchial asthma. The x-ray revealed the source of Robbie's rapid breathing: the lungs were clear, but the heart was quite enlarged. Jenny and Dave were told that Robbie would have to be admitted to the hospital for further tests to find the cause of the enlargement.

Robbie was admitted that evening, a happy, healthy looking baby; and Jenny and Dave remained at his side throughout the night. At first a virus was suspected, but when a recording of the heartbeat was done, the situation proved much more serious: the coronary artery was attached to the pulmonary side of the heart. Robbie was transferred by ambulance to the nearest hospital that performed heart transplants, and the next morning he went into surgery, smiling. The two older boys were sent to stay with a relative temporarily so Jenny and Dave could give all their attention to Robbie. His heart was operated on and he was taken off the bypass machine, but his heart would not begin beating. He was put onto full life-support systems until that afternoon when, miraculously, a heart became available in Texas.

Robbie survived a complete heart transplant, the hospital's 528th and second youngest transplant patient to do so. Surgeons, cardiologists, and nurses told Jenny that it seemed likely that Robbie was thriving because he entered surgery in such good condition. They acknowledged that breastfeeding may have played an important part. Jenny resumed full breastfeeding three days after the transplant when the respirator was removed and Robbie breathed on his own. She continued to breastfeed throughout his three week stay in the hospital and learned that Robbie was the first child known to have been breastfed after a transplant. Because no research had been done on breastfeeding a baby who had had a heart transplant, the surgeon was concerned that Jenny's breast milk might contain immune factors that could cause Robbie's body to reject his new heart. This is the greatest danger faced after a heart transplant. A medical conference was held but no good reason could be found for Jenny to stop breastfeeding, and she was permitted to continue. The physicians' second concern was how to monitor the amount of nourishment Robbie received by breast. It is extremely difficult to measure the amount of milk a breastfed baby receives, so they observed Robbie closely. All outward signs of his health supported Jenny's decision to breastfeed.

Jenny breastfed Robbie day and night, and he had no artificial feeding at the hospital. She carried a beeper that the nurses used to call her every time he was hungry. "My milk would let down each time the beeper went off!" Jenny said. This was inconvenient at times, especially when it went off by mistake, but Jenny was committed to breastfeeding. "I felt that it was the best thing for him. I'd nursed him from birth. I almost lost my milk the first days he was in the hospital because I couldn't nurse. But I kept pumping and telling myself I had to keep my supply up so that when Robbie was able to take my milk, it would be there."

Robbie recovered quite rapidly and without complication. Everyone at the hospital commented on the importance of the special contact that Jenny provided by breastfeeding Robbie in the hospital. Members of the hospital team had warned Jenny prior to the surgery that if Robbie survived, his development would

regress and he would be like a newborn. And just like a newborn, he benefitted from the skin-to-skin contact with his mother.

Today Robbie is eight months old and back at home with his family. It has been four months since the heart transplant, and Robbie is healthy and active again, crawling and standing and beginning to talk. He continues to receive immunosuppressant drugs daily to prevent the rejection of his new heart. He now eats organically grown, commercial baby food but continues to breastfeed as often as he wants. Robbie's breastfeeding and his amazing recovery have been the topic of discussion at many medical conferences and at hospital rounds across the country. Jenny advises any mother whose breastfeeding baby must be hospitalized for any reason to "continue breastfeeding, no matter what it takes. I went through some hard times, and I lost a lot of sleep. You might too, but it is well worth it."

JUANITA'S STORY:
Twins

We met Juanita when her twin boys, José and Pablo, were three and a half weeks old. We had asked a local breastfeeding consultant if there was a mother of twins we could visit. Juanita had said she'd be glad to let us photograph her feeding. We had not been told of any feeding problems before we saw her.

Juanita had had a cesarean section with an epidural anesthetic at term, because she had not been able to find an obstetrician who would deliver her twins vaginally (even though this remains a normal practice in many countries). The babies had been healthy and well nourished in the womb: at birth José had been 6 pounds, 13 ounces and Pablo had been 6 pounds. Juanita had come home from the hospital within a few days. She and her husband had immediately found someone to come and help at the house during the day for the first month, so she could just be with her babies, breastfeed, and try to rest.

She had had lots of support from her local support group for parents of twins and from the mother-to-mother breastfeeding group in her area, The Nursing Mothers Council. In the hospital she had received little help from the staff. She felt this had been due to poor communication between the nurses and herself: "I had a constant battle with the nursery staff," she told us. "They would take the babies away and tell me I needed to rest. Then I would find that the babies had been formula fed in the nursery because the staff had been too busy to bring them back to my room."

Juanita had recovered quickly from her cesarean, but had been quite tired from being up at all hours with José and Pablo. She had tried to sleep as much as she could between feeds. Her husband, Frank, had been very supportive of her breastfeeding and had praised her for her mothering of the boys.

By the time we met Juanita and her babies, José was doing well but Pablo had gained little weight since birth. He was bright and woke regularly for feeds, but Juanita had problems putting him on her breast, and he was often fussy and seemed disinterested in feeding after a short time on the breast. Because he was fussy and José was not, Juanita found herself blaming Pablo at times for his behavior, even though she knew it was not really his fault. When tired and worried because breastfeeding isn't going right, a mother can often blame herself or her baby, not realizing that the problem has to do with the feeding itself.

Both babies had had an episode of thrush at two weeks (probably caused by the antibiotics that Juanita had been given as a matter of routine before her cesarean to prevent postpartum infection from the surgery). Her doctor had planned to treat only the babies, but Juanita had understood that it would be a problem if she got thrush on her nipples, so she had asked for treatment for her nipples too. The thrush had cleared in a week.

Juanita knew about breastfeeding because her mother had breastfed all of her thirteen children. She had the confidence to withstand comments that she got from other people. "I keep getting told not to let them feed longer than twenty minutes," she said. Mothers are often given advice, especially mothers of twins! Juanita had also been told by several people always to feed both babies at the same time so that it would take less time. But she had decided that until breastfeeding was established and both babies were feeding well, she wanted to feed them separately and concentrate on one baby at a time.

First we watched José, the bigger baby, feed. He did well, but we were able to show Juanita how to change the positioning of José's mouth on her breast so he could feed well in less time.

Pablo was the smaller baby, and it was clear that he was one of those small, sleepy babies who needed to have everything in the right place to give him exactly the right stimulus to feed. Several details needed close attention. First, a pillow down behind her back helped Juanita to straighten her posture. This brought her breasts forward and tilted her nipples slightly down, rather than flattening them and tilting the nipples up, the way they had been when she had leaned back. Changing the position of her arms also helped.

She started to feed with Pablo's head in the crook of her arm, but this seemed to give her little control over his head and neck. This is especially important with small babies. We suggested switching arms, putting her baby in the arm opposite from the breast. This way her hand was across his shoulders, cradling his head, allowing Pablo to be well supported along his upper back, neck, and head. Juanita said that she found it easier to help him get well positioned this way. Pablo then needed to be moved quickly onto the breast when he opened his mouth wide.

Juanita also needed to pay special attention to Pablo's lower jaw. It needed to be planted firmly on the underside of her breast as he opened his mouth, so that he took enough of the breast into his mouth.

She did this and Pablo got a good mouthful of breast and started to feed deeply, strongly, and well. He gulped the milk and was finished quite soon, letting his mother know this by coming off the breast. He went onto the other breast after a few tries, and fed deeply and quickly from it too.

While Pablo was learning to go to the breast well, José began to cry loudly, in spite of the fact that he had come off the breast contented not long before. Despite being cuddled he continued crying until his twin brother started to feed well; then José instantly calmed himself.

In the next weeks Juanita found that she still needed practice to get it right, especially with Pablo, but it gradually got better. It got to the point where she was confident enough to feed both babies at the same time when necessary, and Pablo was steadily gaining weight and filling out.

We spoke to Juanita when the twins were seven and a half months old, and both she and the boys were thriving. The boys were good natured and weighed almost 18 pounds each. The pronounced differences in size and development that were so striking when we first saw them, when Pablo was having difficulty at the breast, were gone. Juanita was still breastfeeding, usually feeding both at the same time, which made life simpler for everyone. For the first four months the boys had seldom slept or fed at the same time, meaning Juanita could not count on more than two or three hours of unbroken sleep!

"It's definitely been worth it to breastfeed this long, and I'll continue for as long as we all are enjoying it. It has been difficult," Juanita said, "but what helped me was using a breast pump whenever I needed to leave the boys for an afternoon or when I needed to get four or five hours of unbroken sleep. I rented an electric pump and used the attachment that allowed me to pump both sides at the same time. At times when I did pump I would have to use it every hour or two to keep my supply up. But it worked."

Juanita and the boys did not establish a regular feeding schedule until the twins were seven months old. At four months Juanita had tried giving cereal once a day, hoping it might help them sleep through the night. "The books I'd read said that wouldn't do it; and they were right, it didn't." But the boys, José in particular, enjoyed having a little cereal each morning after feeding, so Juanita continued. At six months José and Pablo started refusing bottles of pumped milk; Juanita felt this was because they liked breastfeeding so much more. They did, however, enjoy drinking a little juice or water from a cup. At seven months they began sleeping through most nights.

Juanita now breastfeeds around 6:30 A.M. and again at 10:00 A.M. The boys also eat a little cereal at one of the morning feeds. They get snacks of fruit or other solid food after their lunch feed and then breastfeed again around 2:30 P.M. If she wants to go out for the afternoon, she leaves them with a baby-sitter who gives them juice or yogurt. Juanita breastfeeds once more in the late afternoon and at that time gives them cereal and a vegetable. Just before bedtime Juanita breastfeeds them once more.

A few weeks ago Juanita thought she might have a breast infection; it was the first problem she had had breastfeeding. One nipple was very sore during feeding. When it didn't clear up after a few days, she went to a clinic and the cause was discovered—a pimple on the nipple. It was recommended that she stop nursing and pump that side until the pimple cleared, but Juanita didn't feel comfortable with the advice. "Once I found out it was not a breast infection and realized that even if the pimple burst the pus would not cause the boys any problems I wasn't concerned." Successful breastfeeding seems to have played a large part in her self-confidence; she knows when to seek advice but feels fully capable of evaluating whatever advice she gets.

KATHY'S STORY:
Inverted Nipple, Large Breasts

Kathy's baby, Sarah, was three months old when we met the family. We had arranged to see them to talk about Kathy's experience of breastfeeding with a very inverted nipple. What we saw was a wonderful example of creativity with breastfeeding when faced with serious difficulty.

Kathy had already breastfed her son, Ben, now eleven years old. After a home birth with no complications, she had started breastfeeding. This had been challenging; her right nipple had been fine, just a bit flat at the beginning. But her left nipple had been turned completely inward. It had not improved at all during pregnancy, when many flat and inverted nipples protrude more because of the hormones of pregnancy.

When she had started breastfeeding, Kathy had tried to feed on the side with the inverted nipple, and found that her baby simply could not manage to take her breast. But Kathy had not been worried. Her mother had been with her to help, and she had had the same problem—with all of her seven healthy breastfed children! She had fed all of them, including twins, on one side only. As the eldest of the family, Kathy had seen this and considered it to be quite normal.

So she had breastfed Ben on one side only, with no supplements until five months. She

had finally stopped breastfeeding altogether at ten months. "I missed it when he stopped," she told us.

Sarah's birth, also at home, had been just as straightforward. Kathy had tried again to breastfeed on the side with the inverted nipple, but had found that it was still not possible. So she had fed on her right side only. She had found that the side she was not using became very engorged (swollen up under her arm), tender, and hot to the touch on the third day after birth, "But I expected it and I knew it would get better. It cleared up by the next day." The side she had been feeding from had not become engorged.

For the first week she had had a sore nipple on the side from which she fed. This, she had realized, was because she had to re-learn positioning. "I also had a very sore back," she remembered, "and I would slump over Sarah as I was feeding her. The sore nipple got better when my back improved and I could sit up in a straighter posture."

Kathy's other challenge was that she had large, soft breasts. But she had discovered that all she had to do was support her breast underneath with one hand throughout the feed. "The only problem is that I can't feed her and do something else at the same time," she told us, "because I need to use both hands. But that means I get to sit down and rest!"

At three months after birth, when we talked, Kathy and Sarah were relaxed and happy with breastfeeding. Sarah would feed for as long as she wanted, and then come off to burp and play for a few minutes. Then she would go back on the same side again for another feed, until she came off herself. "I never tried to time her feeds," Kathy recalled. "My mother never did!"

Kathy had plenty of milk on one side; Sarah fed enthusiastically and well, and came off content. Her weight gain was good, and she was bright and alert. "I am a bit lopsided," Kathy said with a smile. "It took a couple of months for the breast I am not using to stop leaking a lot of milk. Now it leaks just a little, and it is much smaller than the side I do use. But that's not a problem!" Kathy knew that when she stopped breastfeeding, both breasts would end up much the same size (although no woman's two breasts are precisely the same size or shape).

Kathy talked to us about the feelings she had had about her inverted nipple as a teenager. "I thought I was deformed," she said. Although she smiled, it obviously had been a serious concern for her as a very young woman.

She also told us the story of her sister, Frances, who had recently had her first child. Frances had wanted to breastfeed, but she had had very inverted nipples on both sides. In spite of skilled and constant care from Kathy, her mother, and her midwife, Frances had not been able to get her baby to take the breast on either side. "She tried so hard her nipples were sore and bleeding," Kathy told us. "But after three weeks she realized it would not be possible, and decided to pump her breast milk and feed it by bottle." This was a solution that worked for Kathy's sister, even though it was not ideal.

Although many women can breastfeed well with inverted nipples, there are some who simply cannot get the baby to take the breast. Kathy's story of feeding on one side, her mother's story of feeding twins on one side, and her sister's story of pumping and feeding expressed milk were all thoughtful, creative examples of how to overcome serious difficulty.

"I'm so pleased that I've been able to breastfeed," Kathy told us as we left. "It's no trouble when we go out: no bottles of milk. She just feeds quietly under my blouse or a shawl wherever we are. She's a take-along baby!"

Sarah was nine months old when we last spoke to Kathy. Breastfeeding was continuing to go smoothly and there had been no problems. At five and a half months Kathy noticed Sarah was fussy after almost every feed, so she began giving her solid foods at that time. Sarah now takes the breast only once or twice in the morning and once before bed. She's been sleeping through most nights for the past month, but on nights when she does awaken, Kathy breastfeeds her. She plans to continue breastfeeding until Sarah is about a year old.

"The times I breastfeed her are nice and relaxing for both of us. I think I'd miss it if we stopped now. It's the one thing that only I can do for her!"

The Ten Basic Steps:
A Storyboard in English
and Spanish

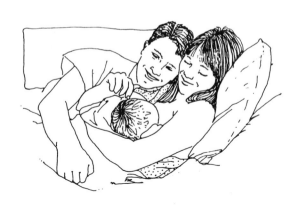

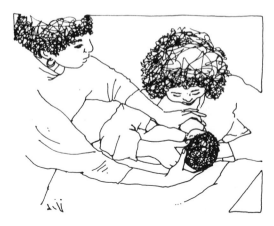

CONCEPT 1:
Breastfeeding is best for women, babies, and families.

CONCEPTO 1:
A dar el pecho o digamos la leche materna es lo mejor para las mujeres, los bebes y las familias.

CONCEPT 2:
It is important to find good, skilled help for the first weeks after the baby is born—to help you get breastfeeding started well, and to help around the house.

CONCEPTO 2:
Después de que nazca el bebé, es muy importante que encuentre a alguien que esta bien cualificada para que le ayude empezar a dar el pecho, y para que le ayude con la limpieza de la casa.

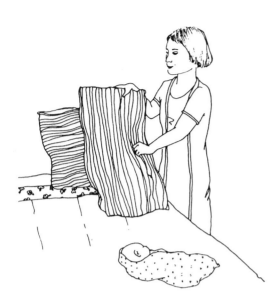

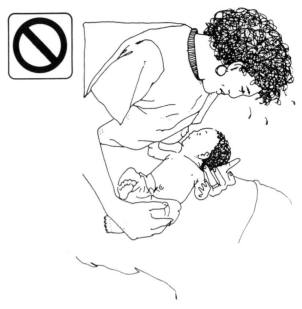

CONCEPT 3:

Before you begin, think about how you feed your baby.

First, you need to get yourself comfortable. Breastfeeding is something that is learned, and like anything you learn it may take time and practice for both you and your baby to do it well.

CONCEPTO 3:

Antes de empezar, piense bien cómo le dara de comer a su bebé.

Primero es necesario que usted este comoda. A dar el pecho es algo que se aprende. Cómo cualquier cosa que se aprende, se necesitara tiempo y practica antes de que su bebé y usted lo hagan bien.

Don't let yourself be in an uncomfortable position when you breastfeed. That will make you tense or tired.

No se ponga en una posición incomoda cuando le esta dando de comer a su bebé. Si esto pasa, se va sentir cansada y tensa.

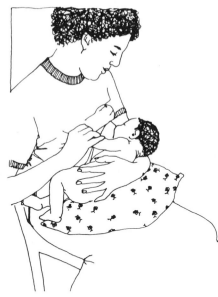

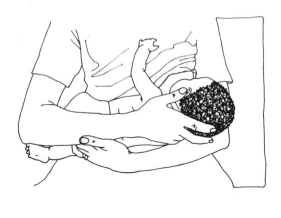

Next, make sure your body is in a good position for feeding—back straight (upright if you are sitting) and your breast free.

Ahora, ponga su cuerpo en una posición buena para dar el pecho-con su espalda recta y con el seno colgando.

Hold your baby very close so the entire front of her body—and her head—are facing you, tucked up next to your body.

Detenga a su bebé bien cerca para que el frente de su cuerpo entero y su cabeza-estan mirando hacia usted, con su cuerpo bien mantenido a un lado del suyo.

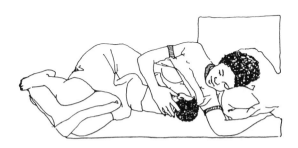

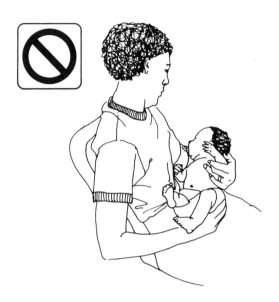

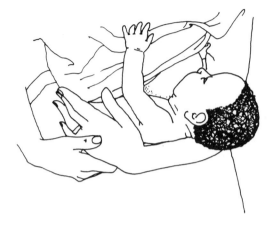

Don't make her have to turn her head to take your breast; it is very difficult for her to feed that way.

No hagas que el bebé tenga que voltear para tomar tu seno, esta posición es muy difícil para que coma el bebé.

Put your baby so that her nose is level with your nipple when her mouth is closed. That way when she takes your breast her lower jaw will be pressed against your breast. If you hold her in your arms, let her head lie on your forearm.

Cuando la boca del bebé esta cerrada, pongalo en una posición en donde su nariz esta al mismo nivel que su pezon. Entonces cuando el bebé toma su seno, la quijada inferior del bebé estara a un lado de tu seno. Si la cabeza del bebé esta reposando sobre su brazo, debe reposar sobre su antebrazo.

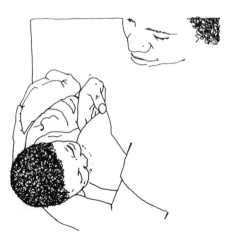

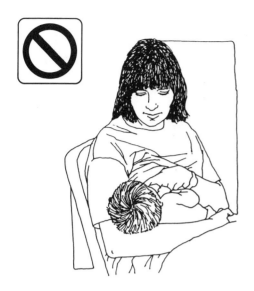

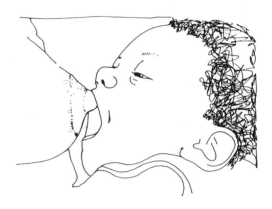

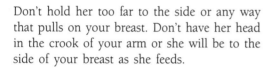

Don't hold her too far to the side or any way that pulls on your breast. Don't have her head in the crook of your arm or she will be to the side of your breast as she feeds.

No detenga al bebé mucho para un lado o en una manera que el pueda arrancar su seno. No ponga la cabeza del bebé en la curva de su brazo porque cuando esta comiendo le arrancara su seno a un lado.

Wait until she gapes her mouth wide open, as if in a yawn, before bringing her on to your breast.

Espere hasta que el bebé tenga su boca bien abierta, así como si estuviera bostezando, antes que usted lo trae a su seno.

Bring the baby to the breast, not the breast to the baby. Don't try to place your breast into her mouth, as if your breast were a bottle; instead, put her onto your breast.

Traiga el bebé a su seno. No trate de poner su seno adentro la boca del bebé, al contrario ponga el bebé sobre el seno.

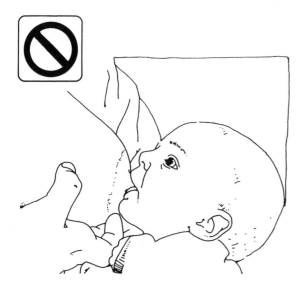

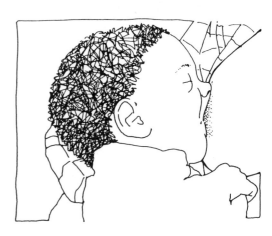

Don't let her just take your nipple in her mouth. It is *breast* feeding, *not* nipple feeding.

Esta actividad se llama "a dar el pecho" no "a dar el pezón." Por eso es importante que el bebé agarre suficiente de su seno en la boca.

If your baby does not take enough breast into her mouth, then gently break the suction, using your finger to release your nipple, and take her off and try again.

Si su bebé no agarra suficiente seno en la boca, con cuidado, use su dedo para sacar el pezón y empieze otra vez.

Make sure she takes a large enough mouthful of breast, not only the nipple. If she takes enough breast into her mouth then your nipple will not get sore.

Cuando el bebé agarra su seno, esté segura que agarro el pezón pero que también agarro suficiente pedazo del seno. Si el bebé toma suficiente bocado de su seno asi no le va doler tanto su pezón y su niño recibera suficiente leche.

Be patient with yourself and with your baby. Take whatever time you both need!

Tenga paciencia con si misma y su bebé. Tomen todo el tiempo que necesitaran para aprender esto.

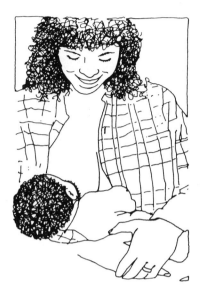

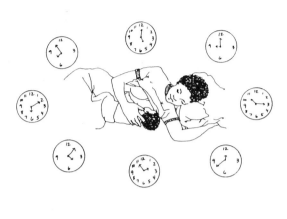

CONCEPT 4:

Breastfeeding should not hurt you! For a while, there may be a quick stab of pain as your baby begins to feed. But if pain continues for more than a few seconds, gently take her off and try again.

CONCEPTO 4:

¡Dando el pecho no debe doler! Al principio usted sentira un poco de dolor. Si el dolor o las molestías siguen por mas de unos segundos, quite el bebé y empieze otra vez.

CONCEPT 5:

Your baby will need to feed often (more often than a baby on artificial milk) throughout the day and also during the night, in the first few weeks. She will not feed at any regular time for a while, but eventually she will settle into a regular schedule.

CONCEPTO 5:

En las primeras semanas, su bebé necesitara comer con mucha frequencía (mas que uno que esta tomando leche artificial) durante el día y también en la noche. No tendra un horario fijo en el principio para comer pero con tiempo se estabilizara.

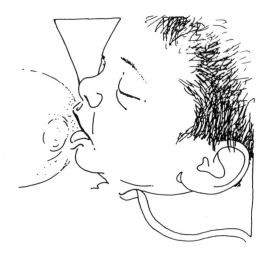
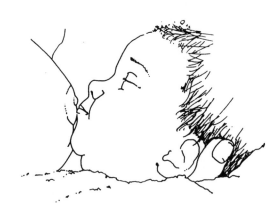

CONCEPT 6:

She will suck deeply and regularly most of the feed and come off the breast by herself when she is finished. Let her show you when she has had enough. Note: Your baby may stop suckling a few times during a feed and then start again. That is normal.

CONCEPTO 6:

El bebé mamara profundamente y con regularidad y dejara de mamar cuando esta lleno. Fijese bien, porque su bebé le enseñara cuando esta lleno. Hay una probabilidad, de vez en cuando, que el bebé se detenga de mamar pero empezara el solo. Esto es normal.

Let your baby come off the breast herself when she has had enough. Don't take her off the breast just because you think the clock tells you she should be done.

Deje que su bebé se quite de su pecho cuando ya ha terminado. No lo quite, porque usted piensa que ya debe de estar lleno.

Remember occasionally to give her the chance to burp/wind after each feed.

Acuerdese de darle una oportunidad a su bebé para que eructa durante o después de cada alimento.

If you or your baby becomes frustrated or upset, stop. Calm yourself. Calm your baby. Then try again.

Si usted o su bebé se siente frustrada o molesta no siga con lo que esta haciendo. Calmese primero. Lluego calme a su bebé. Después trate de empezar otra vez.

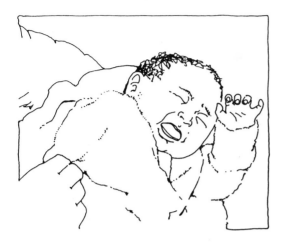

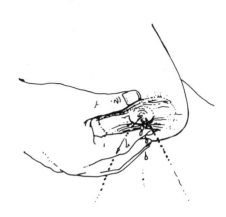

CONCEPT 7:

If your baby cries a lot at the breast—or often cries for a long time after a feeding—or if she does not continue to gain weight, she may not be feeding well. To be sure, first go back over Concepts 2, 3, 4, and 5 and see if you can improve positioning.

If you have a difficult time getting the baby to feed well on your breast, ask someone to look at these pictures and watch you while you put the baby on your breast to see if you are doing everything correctly. Sometimes it is hard to see for yourself, and a helper can be important.

CONCEPTO 7:

Si su bebé esta llorando mucho cuando lo alimenta-o llora a veces después de el alimento-o no esta engordando, puede ser que no esta comiendo bien. Para estar segura, repase los Conceptos 2, 3, 4 y 5 y trate de mejora la posición de su bebé sobre el seno.

Si tiene mucha dificultadidad con esto, preguntarle a alguien que vea estos dibujos mientras la observan dandole el pecho a su bebé, así se dara cuenta si lo esta haciendo bien. A veces es difícil que uno solo vea lo que esta haciendo mal, pero otra persona puede ayudar mucho.

CONCEPT 8:

Learn how to hand express your milk or how to use a breast pump for times when you cannot breastfeed, so that your baby can always have your milk.

CONCEPTO 8:

Aprenda como arrogar leche con su mano o con una pompa a un biberón para que su bebé siempre tenga leche materna para los tiempos cuando usted no le puede dar.

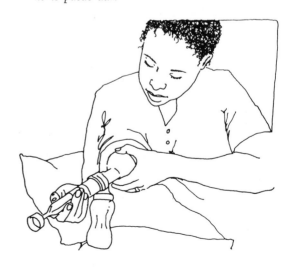

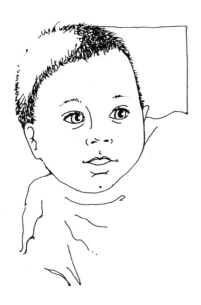

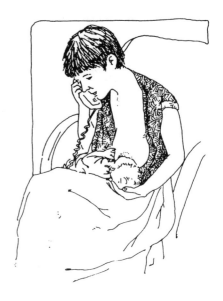

CONCEPT 9:

You will know your baby is thriving if she is gaining weight and looking healthy. If your baby is doing well, she will need no bottles of artificial formula or extra food until at least six months.

CONCEPTO 9:

Usted se dara cuenta si su bebé esta sano porque empezara a aumentar de peso y se vera sano. Si su bebé esta bien, no necesitara leche artificial o otras comidas hasta 6 mes después del naciemiento.

CONCEPT 10:

If you become sick, or if you feel your baby may be sick, *continue giving her your breast milk* and contact a health worker immediately.

CONCEPTO 10:

Si se enferma o siente que su bebé esta enfermo, siga dandole el pecho y hable con una trabajadora de salud inmediatamente.

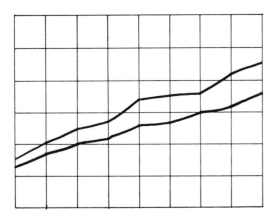

A Final Word

We hope that this book, with its suggestions and stories of breastfeeding women, will help you to breastfeed your baby well and happily. If this book has been helpful, please share it with someone else who might need it. The three of us have learned most of what we know from women like you who have breastfed, and we are confident that women can teach each other about getting breastfeeding right, once they have good information.

The ability to breastfeed is a special and powerful attribute. Breastfeeding well will result in women having increased confidence in themselves and their bodies. We look forward to the future generations of happily breastfed babies and confident breastfeeding women.

About the Authors, Photographer, and Illustrator

Mary Renfrew

Mary Renfrew (formerly known as Mary Houston) is a midwife currently doing research at the National Perinatal Epidemiology Unit, Oxford, England. She was born in 1955 and educated in Scotland, graduating from the University of Edinburgh with a degree in nursing and social science.

As a student she became deeply interested in infant feeding, with a special concern for women who had problems breastfeeding. After

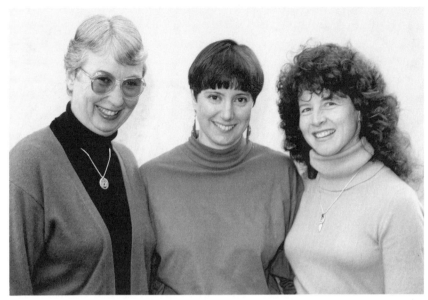

The authors, from left to right: Chloe Fisher, Mary Renfrew, and Suzanne Arms.

qualifying as a midwife, Mary worked with the Medical Research Council in Edinburgh. Here, as part of an interdisciplinary team, she worked on research in breastfeeding, looking at the physiology of breastfeeding and at the problems that mothers and babies have. As a researcher and practitioner, Mary was especially interested in the views and experiences of women, and she found that little of this was reflected in the research that was published in the field. She worked with many breastfeeding mothers during this time, both in the hospital and in the community.

In 1982 she earned her doctorate in Edinburgh for her research in breastfeeding. She wanted to use her skills both to help women and to educate health care practitioners in improving care for women and babies. After working as a midwife in labor and delivery care in Oxford, England, Mary moved to Canada. There she was associate professor in the School of Nursing at The University of Lethbridge, Alberta, for three and a half years. She was also involved with the grassroots midwifery movement in Canada and helped to found the Alberta Association of Midwives, becoming its first spokesperson and Acting President.

In 1987, she returned to the United Kingdom and was appointed to her current position as midwife researcher at the National Perinatal Epidemiology Unit in Oxford. She travels internationally to teach and speak at conferences on midwifery and breastfeeding, and continues to work with mothers and babies. Her aim is to bring together the best of clinical research and clinical practice with women's views of what they need in maternity care.

"I have never felt comfortable with the idea that babies and families are burdens to women that stand in the way of equality. The ability to bear a child and to breastfeed are very powerful, creative aspects of being female. I want to work toward an understanding of how women can have that power recognized and respected."

Chloe Fisher

Chloe Fisher has been a community midwife for more than thirty years. She was born in England in 1932, but spent the years during World War II in foster care in Canada because of the bombings in Britain. Her first training was as a nursery nurse; then she saw a birth, and discovered that she really wanted to be a midwife.

She did the first part of her midwifery training in Cambridge, England, where she worked in a small, midwife-run hospital maternity unit. She learned an enormous amount about breastfeeding there as a result of the good, continuous care given by the midwives. The second part of her training was done in a hospital in Oxford, England, where she saw the impact of artificial and restrictive practices on breastfeeding. When she did community midwifery, caring for women in their homes, she discovered her real love.

In her thirty-two years as a community midwife, Chloe has lost count of the number of mothers and babies for whom she has cared. She knows that by the early 1970s, she had delivered more than one thousand babies. In 1976 she became senior midwife for the Community Midwifery Services in Oxford, the position she still holds. Her work in the community has shown her that childbirth does not do well if rules are imposed, and also that feeding without rules or regulations prevents most breastfeeding problems.

In 1950 she read a pamphlet on feeding called *The Baby Who Does Not Conform to Rules*, which was important in shaping her own attitudes toward breastfeeding. "I've always felt babies should be treated with respect."

Chloe continues to teach midwives and physicians about helping mothers and babies form close relationships, of which breastfeeding is a special part. She now speaks throughout the United Kingdom and internationally and is an adviser to the International Lactation Consultant Association. She served as chair of the committee set up by the Royal College of Midwives in the United Kingdom to investigate the problems of breastfeeding. This committee produced a handbook for midwives, *Successful Breastfeeding*, which is a superb blend of research and clinical wisdom.

Chloe still works day to day with mothers and babies with breastfeeding problems. She wants to continue to work toward women experiencing normal, natural childbirth and enjoying the behavior of the normal newborn who is not subjected to interventions. Her real love is getting mothers and babies together. "This," she says, "is the basis for all my work as a midwife."

Suzanne Arms

Suzanne Arms, the third author, whose photographs also appear throughout this book, was born in New Jersey in 1944. (She is also known by her married name, Suzanne Arms Wimberley.) She graduated from the University of Rochester, New York, in 1965 with honors in literature and a minor in anthropology. Afterward she moved to California, where she taught in day care centers, nursery schools, and Project Head Start, in urban, ghetto, and suburban settings. "I have always been committed to the healing of social ills, but I was an advocate for children long before I understood the relationship between children's and women's issues."

Having grown up during a time in the United States when both natural childbirth and breastfeeding were rare, Suzanne never saw a baby being breastfed until the age of twenty-six, when she was pregnant and living in a Northern California community in which both natural childbirth and breastfeeding were becoming common.

It was the birth of her daughter, Molly, that inspired her to investigate modern childbirth practices. She researched, wrote, and did the photographs for *Immaculate Deception: A New Look at Women and Childbirth*. First published in 1975, it is still in print and is now considered a classic in its field. It is required reading in many college, nursing, and midwifery courses. She has also written *To Love and Let Go* (published in hardback in 1983, and now published in a much expanded and updated paperback edition as *Adoption: A Handful of Hope*). In 1978 she made a childbirth education film, *Five Women, Five Births: A Film About Choices*, which is widely used. Her photographs have appeared in numerous books and publications.

After moving to Palo Alto, California, in 1976, she spearheaded the founding of The Birth Place, a nonprofit group that continues to operate a resource, information, and referral center on birth and parenting, and also a state-licensed childbirth center, near Stanford University. She is also a founding board member of Planetree, a national consumer health organization dedicated to improving hospital care and providing the public with access to medical information so they can be active participants in their own health and medical care. Planetree operates innovative health resource, information, and referral centers in San Francisco and other United States cities and a model hospital unit at Pacific Medical Center in San Francisco and at sites in other cities to assist communities and hospitals in making innovative changes.

As a writer, photographer, and public speaker, she enjoys documenting the pioneering work of those who create positive models for change. Since 1970 she has been an active spokesperson for lay midwifery and home birth.

"Birth, infancy and early childhood experiences create the foundation for our lives. Not only does it affect our physical health and well-being, what we learn during this period of time forms the basis for who we become and how we feel about ourselves and our world. Breastfeeding is simply an integral part of that foundation."

Maggie Conroy

Maggie Conroy is an artist and illustrator who also founded a bookstore within an artists cooperative called the Artifactory, in Palo Alto, California. Today Maggie illustrates books, greeting cards, and birth announcements and also designs flyers.

She was born in Des Moines, Iowa, in 1956, attended Grandview College there, and then moved to Minneapolis and later to California, where she earned a master's degree in art therapy from the College of Notre Dame in 1983. Her first job was as an art therapist at Mills–Peninsula Hospital, near San Francisco, where she worked with preadolescent children with emotional difficulties, and with their parents. She also worked in several preschools in the San Francisco Bay area, including the Apple Childcare Center, which Apple Computer set up for the young children of its employees.

"As a preschool teacher I saw the concerns and challenges mothers faced in balancing child rearing, family, and work. In my work as a teacher and as an artist, I try to find ways to communicate understanding and support for the difficult balance women today must maintain between their roles as mother and as worker."

This book is a blend of all of our experiences and backgrounds, and we are certain that no one of us could have written it without each of the others. Our goal has been to put into writing, photographs, and drawings the experience and knowledge we all have. Mary's writing skill, combined with academic knowledge and clinical understanding, Chloe's hands-on wisdom, Suzanne's understanding of women's needs, plus her extraordinary skill as a photographer and writer, together with Maggie's accurate and evocative drawings, made it possible to put together a book that is different from anything that has come before.

Learning about breastfeeding today, after so much knowledge and understanding has been lost through the years, it is not easy. We learned about breastfeeding by talking and working with mothers through many years (we have a total of seventy years' experience among us!), from personal experiences of breastfeeding, and from reading about and studying the subject. We have also learned from each other in the course of writing. This book includes all of our approaches, and what it contains is what we all believe to be true.

Our plan was to write a clear, basic guide for women on how to get breastfeeding right and how to solve problems, with accurate information and pictures. We believe there is new and useful information in this book for everyone. If you find any parts especially helpful, or especially unhelpful, we would like to know. Please write to us, care of our publisher. This will help us improve the book in future editions.

Where to Find Help

You will find this list of addresses helpful if you want to contact groups that assist breastfeeding women. It is as up-to-date as we can make it. Some names and addresses may not be current by the time you read this book. We apologize if you have difficulty contacting any of them. Please let us know if this happens!

If you help to organize any of these groups and find that we have given an old address, please write to us in care of our publishers so we can update our list.

We know that there are many groups that help breastfeeding women that we have not listed for lack of space. The addresses listed here are to get you started. These groups will be able to put you in touch with local groups. If you know of a group in an area that we have not listed, please write to us.

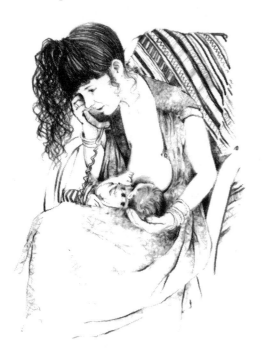

Some of these are support groups for breast-feeding mothers, some are educational groups, and others are political pressure groups, such as International Baby Food Action Network (IBFAN). Any group will put you in touch with local breastfeeding support if they cannot give you help directly.

The list begins with international groups. Following these, the addresses are grouped by region or continent, and then broken down by country. Addresses for groups in the United Kingdom and the United States that assist parents of babies with special needs follow the general list. Closing this section are national and international addresses for companies you can write or call for information on renting or purchasing breast pumps.

International

International Childbirth Education Association
P.O. Box 20048
Minneapolis, MN 55420
United States
Tel. (612) 854-8660

International Lactation Consultants
  Association
P.O. Box 4031
University of Virginia Station
Charlottesville, VA 22903
United States

La Leche League International (LLLI)
P.O. Box 1209
Franklin Park, IL 60131-8209
United States
Tel. (800) LA LECHE

UNICEF
Margaret Kyenkya
Project Officer, Infant Feeding
3 United Nations Plaza
New York, NY 10017
United States
Tel. (212) 326-7000

Africa

EGYPT

Society of Friends of Breastfeeding
26A El Gazira Alwosta St.
Zamalek
Cairo
Egypt

KENYA

IBFAN Africa
P.O. Box 34308
Nairobi
Kenya
Tel. (2) 334 638

Breastfeeding Information Group
P.O. Box 59436
Nairobi
Kenya

SOUTH AFRICA

National Childbirth and Parenting Association
70 Ennisdale Dr.
Durban North 4051
South Africa

SWAZILAND

Swaziland Infant Nutrition
Action Network
P.O. Box 1032
Mbabane
Swaziland

Caribbean

BERMUDA

Susan Kessaren
P.O. Box HM 1214
Hamilton
HMFX
Bermuda

DUTCH ANTILLES

Fundashion Leche di Mama
c/o Martha Wansing
P.O. Box 2043
Brakke Put Abou 100
Curacao
Dutch Antilles

TRINIDAD

IBFAN Caribbean
P.O. Box 410
Port of Spain
Trinidad and Tobago

The Informative Breastfeeding Service (TIBS)
16 Gray St.
St. Clair
Port of Spain
Trinidad W.I.

Central and South America

ARGENTINA

Nunu - Association de Ayuda
Materna
Av. San Martin 1450
1638 Vicente Lopez (Bs. As.)
Republica Argentina

COLOMBIA

UNICEF Oficina Regional Para America
    Latina y El Caribe
Juan R. Aguilar, Senior Regional Advisor
Primary Health Care
Carrera 13 No. 75-74
Bogotá, Colombia

(This office is the location for information on a project called "Kangaroo Baby," which puts premature infants in skin-to-skin contact with their mothers as many hours a day as possible.)

COSTA RICA

IBFAN/CEFEMINA
Apartado 949
San Jose 1000
Costa Rica
Tel. (2) 44620

ECUADOR

IBFAN South America
c/o CEPAM
Apartado 182-C Suc 15
Quito
Ecuador

PERU

Comite Pervano Pro-alimentatcion
Infantil
Apartado 949
Lima 100
Peru

East Asia

SOUTH KOREA

IBFAN East Asia
c/o Citizen's Alliance for Consumer Protection
    (CACPK)
K.P.O. Box 411
Seoul 110
South Korea

Europe

EUROPEAN OFFICE

IBFAN/GIFA
P.O. Box 157
1211 Geneva 19
Switzerland
Tel. (22) 98 9164

BELGIUM

V.Z.W. Borstvoeding Belgie
c/o Els Flies
Cardijnstraat 36
2190 Essen (Wildert)
Belgium

Regionale Stillgruppe des deuschsprachigen
    gebeites Belgiens
c/o Juliet Elsen
Kinkebahn 120
4731 Eynatten
Belgium

Brussels Childbirth Trust (English and
    French speaking)
Av. Hebron 136
1950 Kraainem
Belgium

DENMARK

Britta Mathiasen
Granlunden 93
6700 Esbjerg
Denmark

FINLAND

Ensi-ja Turvakotien liito
Museo Kato 24A
00100 Helsinki
Finland

FRANCE

Action pour Allaitement
19, rue de Dalhain
67200 Strasbourg
France

Message
16 Bis Rue do Cergy
Neuville sur Oise
N5000 Cergy
France

HUNGARY

Dr. Eszter Bonta
1 Pagony St.
1124 Budapest
Hungary

IRELAND

Irish Childbirth Trust
Methodist House
Roscrea
Co. Tipperary
Ireland

MALTA

Malta Breastfeeding Mothers
c/o Marianna Theuma
5 Trafalgar Flats
Cardinal St.
Vittoriose
Malta

NETHERLANDS

Vereniging Borstvoeding Natuurlijk
Postbus 119
3960 BC Wijk bij Duurstede
Netherlands

NORWAY

Ammehjelpen
St. Olavsgate 5
Oslo 1
Norway

POLAND

Polish Breastfeeding Support Group
c/o Ewa Nitecka Lachmama 2 m 65
02-786 Warsawa
Poland

SWEDEN

Amningshjalpen
Kvinnocentrum
Biger Jarlsg. 22
114 34
Stockholm
Sweden

UNITED KINGDOM

Association of Breastfeeding Mothers
10 Hershell Rd.
London SE 23 1EG
United Kingdom
Tel. (01) 778 4769

Breastfeeding Promotion Group
National Childbirth Trust
Alexandra House
Oldham Terrace
Acton
London W3 6NH
United Kingdom
Tel. (01) 992 8637

La Leche League of Great Britain
BM 3424
London WC1 6XX
United Kingdom
Tel. (01) 242 1278

WEST GERMANY

Arbeitsgemeinschaft freir Stillgruppen
c/o Sylvia Brunn
Rheingaustr 14
5420 Welterod
West Germany

Middle East

ISRAEL

Israel Childbirth Education Centre
P.O. Box 3731
Haifa 31037
Israel

JORDAN

IBFAN Middle East
c/o UNICEF Regional Office
P.O. Box 811721
Amman
Jordan

North America

CANADA

IBFAN NORTH AMERICA/INFACT CANADA
10 Trinity Square
Toronto
Ontario
Canada
Tel. (416) 595–5819

CANADA FRANCAIS

Secretariat General de la Leche League
CF. P. 874
Ville St.-Laurent
Quebec H4L 4W3
Canada

Health and Welfare Canada
Child and Family Health Programs/Health
  Promotion Directorate
Jeanne Mance Bldg., Fourth Floor
Tunney's Pasture
Ottawa
Ontario K1A 1B4
Canada
Tel. (613) 996-1125

UNITED STATES

ACTION for Corporate Accountability
  (IBFAN)
3255 Hennepin Ave. S.
Suite 255
Minneapolis, MN 55408
United States
Tel. (612) 823-1571

(See also International. La Leche League International (LLLI) has branches in each state.)

Nursing Mothers Counsel, Inc.
P.O. Box 50063
Palo Alto, CA 94303
United States

(Based primarily in the San Francisco Bay Area. Hotline numbers are listed in local telephone directories.)

South Central Asia

INDIA

IBFAN South Central Asia
c/o Anil Saxena
Punjab National Bank
Vasco de Gama
Goa
India

MAURITIUS

Mauritian Action for the Promotion of
  Breastfeeding and Infant
Nutrition (MAPBIN)
P.O. Box 1134
Port Louis
Mauritius

South East Asia

MALAYSIA

Annalies and Jean-Pierre Allain
IOCU
P.O. Box 1045
10830 Penang
Malaysia
Tel. (4) 366506

PHILIPPINES

IBFAN/BUNSO
6B, K-6th Street
Kamias Road
Quezon City
Philippines

GABRIELA, Commission on Health
Edith Espino
1832 UP Bliss
Diliman
Quezon City
Philippines

Nursing Mothers Association of the
    Philippines
Bldg. 24, Apt. 43
Bliss
Pagassa
Quezon City
Philippines

SINGAPORE

Singapore Breastfeeding Mothers Group
c/o Consumers Association of Singapore
NTUC Annexe
Shenton Way
Singapore 0106

South Pacific

AUSTRALIA

Nursing Mothers Association of Australia
5 Glendale St.
Nunawading 3131
Australia
Tel. (03) 877 5011

International Breastfeeding Affiliation
13 Glen St.
Hawthorn
Victoria 3122
Australia

NEW ZEALAND

IBFAN South Pacific
New Zealand Coalition for Trade and
    Development
P.O. Box 11345
Wellington
New Zealand
(04) 851909

PAPUA NEW GUINEA

Susu Mamas
P.O. Box 5857
Brooko
Port Moresby
Papua New Guinea

VANUATU

Mama Blong Vanuatu
P.O. Box 819
Port Vila
Vanuatu

Groups that Assist
Parents of Babies with
Special Needs

UNITED KINGDOM

Association for Spina Bifida and Hydrocephalus
22 Upper Woburn Place
London WC1H OEP
United Kingdom
Tel. (01) 388 1382

Cleft Lip and Palate Association (CLAPA)
Hospitals for Sick Children
Great Ormond St.
London WC1N 3JH
United Kingdom
Tel. (01) 405 9200

Down's Syndrome Association
First Floor
12-13 Clapham Common South Side
London SW4 7AA
United Kingdom
Tel. (01) 720 0008

In Touch
10 Norman Rd.
Sale
Cheshire M33 3DF
United Kingdom
Tel. (061) 962 4441

(This is an organization that puts parents in touch with others who are caring for a similarly handicapped child. They publish a newsletter, giving information on organizations and literature. National and overseas membership.)

National Association for Parents of
   Prematures (NIPPERS)
c/o Caroline Kerr-Smith
49 Allison Rd.
Acton
London W3 6HZ
United Kingdom
Tel. (01) 992 9310

UNITED STATES

American Cleft Palate Foundation
1218 Grandview Ave.
Pittsburgh, PA 15211
United States
Tel. (800) 242-5338

National Down's Syndrome Congress (NDSC)
1800 Dempster St.
Park Ridge, IL 60068-1146
United States
Tel. (800) 232-6372

Breast Pump & Breastfeeding Supplementer Manufacturers

Ameda AG
Baarerstrasse 75
CH6300 Zug 2
Switzerland
Tel. (42) 23 4353

Ameda/Egnell Inc.
765 Industrial Dr.
Cary, IL 60013
United States
Tel. (800) 323-8750

Egnell Ameda Ltd.
Medical Equipment
Quarry House
Mill Lane
Uckfield
East Sussex
TN22 5AA
United Kingdom
(08) 256 7715

Egnell-Ameda Medical Inc.
3 Vista Dr.
Fonthill
Ontario LOS 1E2
Canada
Tel. (416) 892-5343

(Ameda has offices throughout the world. The home office in Switzerland can provide addresses for those countries not listed here.)

Medela AG
Lattichstrasse 4
6340 Baar
Switzerland
Tel. (42) 31 1616

Medela Inc.
P.O. Box 386
6711 Sands Rd.
Crystal Lake, IL 60014
United States
Tel. (800) 435-8316 (toll free) or
   (815) 455-6920 (collect calls)

(Medela has offices throughout the world. The home office in Switzerland can provide addresses for those countries not listed here.)

National Childbirth Trust
Alexandra House
Oldham Terrace
Acton
London W3 6NH
United Kingdom
Tel. (01) 992 8637

(Ameda cylinder pump is available from National Childbirth Trust.)

Trudell Inc.
P.O. Box 382
926 Leathorne St.
London
Ontario N6A 4W1
Canada
Tel. (519) 685-8800

(Trudell Inc. is the Medela distributor for Canada.)

Lact-Aid Inernational Inc.
Dept. BSB
P.O. Box 1066
Athens, TN 37303
United States

(This is the manufacturer of a nursing supplementer. Medela makes a version of a supplementer too.)

Books You Might
Find Helpful

Some of you may like more detail on specific aspects of breastfeeding than we have been able to provide in this book. This is a short list of books that you might find helpful.

Balancing Acts: On Being a Mother, Katherine Gieve, ed. (London: Virago, 1989). If you want to know how other women feel about being mothers and the challenges of mothering in Western culture, this book will interest you. It is a collection of women's accounts, telling their experiences and feelings.

Born Too Early: Special Care for Your Preterm Baby, Margaret Redshaw, Rodney Rivers, and Deborah Rosenblatt (Oxford, New York, and Toronto: Oxford University Press, 1985). This book will be helpful to anyone who has a preterm baby. It has a good section on breastfeeding and on caring for yourself and your family.

Breastfeeding Matters, Maureen Minchin (Melbourne, Australia: Alma Publications/George Allen and Unwin, 1985). This book is a good review of the practical problems and the politics of infant feeding. It is well referenced and full of facts on all aspects of breastfeeding: nutrition, allergies, culture, and practical aspects such as positioning. Available in North America through Birth and Life Bookstore, P.O. Box 70625, Seattle, WA 98107 (telephone: (206) 789–4444); in the United Kingdom through the National Childbirth Trust (see address in "Where to Find Help"); or direct from Alma Publications, 5 St. George's Rd., Armadale, Victoria, Australia.

Crying Baby, Sleepless Nights, Sandy Jones (New York: Warner Books, 1983). Dedicated to "all the mothers who are reading this book at 4 A.M., and to all the babies who long not to have to cry anymore." This book will be a good, practical support for anyone with an inconsolable baby.

Drugs, Vitamins, Minerals in Pregnancy, Ann K. Henry and Jil Feldhausen (Tucson, AZ: Fisher Books, 1989). This is a new, easy-to-read book, listing the commonly used drugs or medications and their possible side effects when taken during pregnancy or lactation. It can be obtained directly through Fisher Books, P.O. Box 38040, Tucson, AZ 85740–8040.

Hi Mom! Hi Dad!: The First Twelve Months of Parenthood (101 cartoons), Lynn Johnston (Toronto: Stoddart Publishing Co., 1985). These wonderful cartoons will entertain you and at the same time reassure you that life with a new baby is a mixture of joy, frustration, and exhaustion. An important book to keep you balanced and laughing with your new baby around.

Nursing Mother's Companion, Kathleen Huggins (Boston: Harvard Common Press, 1986). We recommend this book's section on working outside the home and breastfeeding called "Traveling Together, Being Apart." It gives practical suggestions on how to breastfeed while being separated from your baby, and summarizes the types of breast pumps that are available, discussing the advantages and disadvantages of each.

Nursing Your Baby with a Cleft Lip or Palate, Sarah Coulter Danner and Edward Cerutti (1984). This small, inexpensive pamphlet contains information and illustrations on breastfeeding a baby with a cleft lip or palate. The pamphlet is available from the Childbirth Graphics Association, 1210 Culver Rd., Rochester, NY 14609.

Nursing Your Baby with Down's Syndrome, Sarah Coulter Danner and Edward Cerutti (1984). This inexpensive pamphlet tells how to breastfeed a baby with Down's syndrome. Contains illustrations. You can obtain the pamphlet by writing to Childbirth Graphics Association (address listed in the previous entry).

The Politics of Breastfeeding, Gabrielle Palmer (London, Sydney, and Wellington: Pandora, 1988). An excellent discussion of the problems women face today. It covers political, economic, and cultural issues. Essential reading for anyone concerned with worldwide issues in breastfeeding.

A Practical Guide to Breastfeeding, Jan Riordan (St. Louis, Toronto, and London: C. V. Mosby Co., 1983). Written for health workers, this book provides answers to some of the more obscure problems. Widely referenced.

Shared Parenthood: A Handbook for Fathers, Johanna Roeber (London, Melbourne, and Auckland: Century Paperbacks, 1987). A well-written, sensible, and caring book about pregnancy, birth, and infant care from the father's point of view. Good discussions of men's feelings about breastfeeding.

World of the Newborn, Martin Richards (New York: Harper & Row, 1980). This book will tell you about a newborn baby's amazing range of abilities and will provide a general understanding of babies.

The authors have produced audio-visual materials related to "Bestfeeding." To find out about these educational videos, posters, etc., contact the following distributors:

UNITED STATES

Cesarean Prevention Movement (CPM)
1008 Westcott Street
Syracuse, NY 13210
Tel. (315) 424-1942

AUSTRALIA

The Lactation Resource Center
c/o The Nursing Mothers Association of
   Australia
P.O. Box 231
Nunawading 3131
Victoria
Australia

UNITED KINGDOM

National Childbirth Trust (NCT)
Alexandra House
Oldham Terrace
Acton, London W3 6NH
United Kingdom
Tel. (01) 992 8637

GLOSSARY: AN EXPLANATION OF TERMS USED IN THIS BOOK

Anesthesia. *See* General, Epidural, Regional, or Spinal anesthesia.

Areola. The circular, dark area around the nipples.

Breast abscess. An infected area in the breast that is swollen and tender and filled with pus. *See page 127.*

Breast pump. A device that helps extract milk from the breast. It works by suction and can be powered by hand, by battery, or by electricity. *See pages 89–91.*

Breast shells. Pieces of curved plastic or glass that fit inside the bra. Also called *milk cups*. It is claimed that they pull out inverted nipples, though this has never been proven. Some types can be used to collect excess breast milk.

Burping. Bringing up gas or wind.

Candida. *See* Thrush.

Colostrum. The thick, yellow milk produced in the first few days of breastfeeding. It is high in protein and protects the baby from infection. *See page 76.*

Demand feeding. *See* Flexible feeding.

Engorgement. Painful swelling of the breasts. *See pages 123–124.*

Epidural anesthesia. Anesthesia given to help delivery via a tube into the back. It numbs from the waist to the thighs and does not put the woman to sleep. It can be used to assist a normal or a cesarean section delivery. *See page 32.*

Flat nipples. *See* Nonprotractile nipples.

Flexible feeding. Feeding a baby when the mother and child decide the time is right rather than by a set schedule. Some people call this *demand feeding*; we prefer to think of it as feeding that suits both the mother and baby (flexible) rather than feeding that is demanded by the baby. *See page 79.*

Foremilk. The milk that the baby takes during the first few minutes of feeding. It has a high volume (good for the baby's fluid intake) and has a low fat concentration. A baby needs a balance of both foremilk and hindmilk.

General anesthetic. Anesthetic that puts a woman into a special state of consciousness to help either a cesarean section delivery or with complications of vaginal birth, such as retained afterbirth. *See page 32.*

Hindmilk. The milk that a baby takes after the first few minutes of feeding. It is lower in volume (so the feeding slows down) and higher in calories or fat (good for the baby's growth and energy level). A baby needs a good intake of both hindmilk and foremilk. *See pages 76–79.*

Inverted nipples. A nipple that turns inward rather than projecting outward, resembling a small crater. One or both nipples may be inverted. *See pages 95-97.*

Jaundice. A condition, quite common in the first few days after birth, where the baby's skin and eyes become yellow. Because it occurs for a number of reasons, it is important to discover the particular cause for each baby. *See pages 145–147.*

Letdown reflex. The breasts' release of milk for the baby. Some women experience it as a tingling sensation. It is caused by the hormone oxytocin. *See page 73.*

Lochia. The loss of blood a woman experiences after the birth of a baby that continues for the first few weeks. Breastfeeding speeds up the process, so the flow is heavier but stops sooner. *See page 73.*

Mastitis. Red, inflamed breasts. *See pages 124–126.*

Milk ejection reflex. *See* Letdown reflex.

Nipple shields. Thin, plastic shapes that fit over the nipple to offer protection from pain when the baby feeds. They can reduce the milk supply and can cause other problems. They are helpful in the long term in only a few situations.

Nonprotractile nipples. Flat nipples that will not project outward. *See pages 95–97.*

Oxytocin. The hormone released when a baby feeds or when the mother thinks about feeding. It causes the milk to be released (the letdown reflex). It is also released when a woman makes love. Synthetic preparations of this hormone, used to induce or to accelerate labor, are marketed as Pitocin or as Syntocinon. *See page 73.*

Prolactin. The hormone released when feeding a baby that causes the breasts to produce more milk. It plays an important part in the supply and demand mechanism. *See page 71.*

Regional anesthesia. This term covers both epidural and spinal anesthesia. *See* the listings for these terms.

Spinal anesthesia. Anesthesia that numbs the lower part of the body but does not put the individual to sleep. It is administered via a needle into the back.

Thrush. An infection that occurs most commonly in the vagina or in a baby's mouth and digestive system. Also known as *candida* or *yeast infection*. It is caused by an overabundance of yeasts that are normally present in the body. Symptoms are a white discharge in the vagina or white flecks on a baby's tongue and cheeks. *See pages 130–131.*

Yeast infection. *See* Thrush.

BIBLIOGRAPHY

The information in this book is based on extensive reading of research as well as on clinical experience. We have read and reviewed hundreds of books and articles; this listing contains some of the work that has been most helpful.

Ardran, G. M., F. H. Kemp, and J. Lind. "A Cineradiographic Study of Bottle Feeding." *British Journal of Radiology* 31 (1958): 11–12.

———"A Cineradiographic Study of Breast-feeding." *British Journal of Radiology* 31 (1958): 156–162.

Auerbach, K. G., and L. M. Gartner. "Breastfeeding and Human Milk: Their Association with Jaundice in the Neonate." *Clinics in Perinatology* 14, no. 1 (1987): 89–107.

Colebunders, R., et al. "Breastfeeding and Transmission of HIV." [letter] *Lancet* 2, no. 8626 (1988): 1487.

Department of the Environment, Central Directorate of Environmental Protection. "Dioxins in the Environment." Pollution paper no. 27. HMSO: London (1989).

European Collaborative Study. "Mother-to-Child Transmission of HIV Infection." *Lancet* 2, no. 8619 (1988): 1039–1042.

Garza, C., R. J. Schanler, N. F. Butte, and K. J. Motil. "Special Properties of Human Milk." *Clinics in Perinatology* 14, no. 1 (1987): 11–32.

Gunther, M. *Infant Feeding.* London: Methuen, 1971.

Hall, B. "Changing Composition of Milk and Early Development of an Appetite Control." *Lancet* 1, no. 7910 (1975): 779–781.

Hytten, F. "Clinical Studies in Lactation, II: Variations in the Major Constituents During a Feeding." *British Medical Journal* 1 (1954): 176–179.

Illingworth, R. S., and D. G. H. Stone. "Self-Demand Feeding in a Maternity Unit." *Lancet* 1, no. 14 (1952): 683–687.

Inch, S., and S. Garforth. "Establishing and Maintaining Lactation." In *Effective Care in Pregnancy and Childbirth*, ed. I. Chalmers, M. Enkin, and M. J. N. C. Kierse. Oxford: Oxford University Press, 1989.

Inch, S., and M. J. Renfrew. "Common Breastfeeding Problems." In *Effective Care in Pregnancy and Childbirth*, ed. I. Chalmers, M. Enkin, and M. J. N. C. Kierse. Oxford: Oxford University Press, 1989.

Italian Multicentre Study. "Epidemiology, Clinical Features, and Prognostic Factors of Paediatric HIV Infection." *Lancet* 2, no. 8619 (1988): 1043–1046.

Lepage, P., et al. "Postnatal Transmission of HIV from Mother to Child." [letter] *Lancet* 2, no. 8555 (1987): 400.

Lissauer, T. "Impact of AIDS on Neonatal Care." *Archives of Disease in Childhood* 64 (1989): 4–7.

Martin, J., and A. White. *Infant Feeding: 1985 Office of Population Censuses and Surveys.* London: Her Majesty's Stationery Office, 1988.

McNeilly, A. S., I. C. Robinson, M. J. Houston, and P. W. Howie. "Release of Oxytocin and Prolactin in Response to Suckling." *British Medical Journal* 286 (1983): 257–259.

Meier, P. "Bottle and Breast Feeding: Effects on Transcutaneous Oxygen Pressure and Temperature in Preterm Infants." *Nursing Research* 37 (1988): 36–41.

Meier, P., and G. Cranston-Anderson. "Responses of Small Preterm Infants to Bottle- and Breastfeeding." *Maternal and Child Nursing* 12 (1987): 97–105.

Minchin, M. *Breastfeeding Matters.* Melbourne, Australia: Alma Publications/George Allen and Unwin, 1985.

Nutrition Committee of the Canadian Paediatric Society and the Committee of Nutrition of the American Academy of Pediatrics. "Breast-Feeding: A Commentary in Celebration of the International Year of the Child." *Pediatrics* 62 (1978): 591–601.

Royal College of Midwives. *Successful Breastfeeding: A Practical Guide for Midwives and Others Supporting Breastfeeding Mothers.* London: Royal College of Midwives, 1988.

Salariya, E. M., P. M. Easton, and J. I. Cater. "Duration of Breast-Feeding After Early Initiation and Frequent Feeding." *Lancet* 2, no. 8100 (1978): 1141–1143.

Senturia, Y. D., et al. "Breast-Feeding and HIV Infection." [letter] *Lancet* 2, no. 8555 (1987): 400–401.

Stanback, M., et al. "Breastfeeding and HIV Transmission in Haitian Children." Paper presented at the 4th International Conference on AIDS, Stockholm, 1988.

Thapa, S., R. V. Short, and M. Potts. "Breastfeeding, Birth Spacing and Their Effects on Child Survival." *Nature* 335 (1988): 679–682.

Thomsen, A. C., et al. "Course and Treatment of Milk Stasis, Non-Infectious Inflammation of the Breast and Infectious Mastitis in Nursing Women." *American Journal of Obstetrics and Gynecology* 149, no. 5 (1984): 492–495.

Uvnas-Moberg, K. "The Gastrointestinal Tract in Growth and Reproduction." *Scientific American,* July 1989, 78–83.

Verronen, P. "Breastfeeding: Reasons for Giving Up and Transient Lactational Crises." *Acta Pediatrica Scandinavica* 71 (1982): 447–450.

Widstrom, A. M., et al. "Gastric Suction in Healthy Newborn Infants." *Acta Pediatrica Scandinavica* 76 (1987): 566–572.

Woolridge, M. W. "The Anatomy of Infant Sucking, and the Aetiology of Sore Nipples." *Midwifery* 2 (1986): 164–176.

Woolridge, M. W., J. D. Baum, and R. F. Drewett. "Individual Patterns of Milk Intake During Breastfeeding." *Early Human Development* 7 (1982): 265–272.

Woolridge, M. W., and C. Fisher. "Colic, 'Overfeeding,' and Symptoms of Lactose Malabsorption in the Breast-Fed Baby: A Possible Artifact of Feed Management?" *Lancet* 2, no. 8607 (1988): 382–384.

Ziegler, J. B., et al. "Postnatal Transmission of AIDS-Associated Retrovirus from Mother to Infant." *Lancet* 1, no. 8434 (1985): 896–899.

INDEX OF COMMONLY
ASKED QUESTIONS

INDEX OF
WORDS AND PHRASES

Superwoman myth, 26
Supplemental feeding
  case study, 171–174
  milk supply and, 134
Support
  See also Helpers
  emotional, 21–23
  for expressing milk, 90, 92
  importance of, 28
  practical, 21–23
  for sick mother, 99
  skilled assistance, 21, 25
  sources of, 201–208, 210
  types of help needed, 21
Support groups, 24
  for adoptive mothers, 107
  electric pumps rented by, 90
  for parents of special-needs babies, 100–101, 207
  for problem solving, 114
Swaddling, as crying remedy, 139

T

Taking care of yourself, 25–26, 86, 98
Teats, nipples vs., 166
Tension, milk release and, 74
Things to avoid, 65, 79
Thrush, 130–131
  as antibiotic side effect, 126
  in case study, 181
  defined, 212
Timing. *See* Frequency of breastfeeds; Length of breastfeeds
Too little/too much milk. *See* Milk supply
Too much milk, 122, 136–137, 175–176
Triplets, 9, 73
Tube feeding, 105
Twins, 9

See also Multiple births
  case study, 180–182
  first feedings of, 46
  milk supply and, 72–73

U

UNICEF, 202
Urine, indications of health in, 87
Uterine contractions, breastfeeding and, 8

V

Vegetarian diet, 97
Visualization, milk release and, 74
Vitamin C, 116
Vomit, blood in, 129, 147

W

Warm compresses
  for engorgement, 124
  as home remedy, 115
  milk release and, 74
Water. *See* Fluids
Weaning, 109–111
  breast abscess and, 127
  myth and reality, 167
Weight loss in baby
  case study, 169–170
  health care warning for, 117
Weight loss in mother, 8, 97
White spots on baby's mouth, 130
White spots on nipples, 126
Working mother, 11–12
  bottle feeding and, 151
  breastfeeding problems and, 154–155
  case study, 171–173
  expressing milk by, 11, 89–94, 155
World Health Organization, artificial milk marketing code by, 159